Science of Spices and Culinary Herbs

Latest Laboratory, Pre-clinical, and Clinical Studies

(*Volume 2*)

Edited by

Atta-ur-Rahman, *FRS*

Kings College, University of Cambridge, Cambridge, UK

M. Iqbal Choudhary

&

Sammer Yousuf

H.E.J. Research Institute of Chemistry, International Center for Chemical and Biological Sciences, University of Karachi, Karachi, Pakistan

Science of Spices & Culinary Herbs

Latest Laboratory, Pre-clinical, and Clinical Studies

Volume # 2

Editors: Atta-ur-Rahman, M. Iqbal Choudhary, and Sammer Yousuf

ISSN (Online): 2590-0781

ISSN (Print): 2590-0773

ISBN (Online): 978-981-14-4149-3

ISBN (Print): 978-981-14-4147-9

ISBN (Paperback): 978-981-14-4148-6

©2020, Bentham Books imprint.

Published by Bentham Science Publishers Pte. Ltd. Singapore. All Rights Reserved.

need for a court order if at any point you breach any terms of this License Agreement. In no event will any delay or failure by Bentham Science Publishers in enforcing your compliance with this License Agreement constitute a waiver of any of its rights.

3. You acknowledge that you have read this License Agreement, and agree to be bound by its terms and conditions. To the extent that any other terms and conditions presented on any website of Bentham Science Publishers conflict with, or are inconsistent with, the terms and conditions set out in this License Agreement, you acknowledge that the terms and conditions set out in this License Agreement shall prevail.

Bentham Science Publishers Pte. Ltd.
80 Robinson Road #02-00
Singapore 068898
Singapore
Email: subscriptions@benthamscience.net

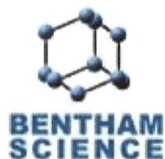

BENTHAM SCIENCE

CONTENTS

PREFACE

Spices and culinary herbs have been in use since ancient times for medicinal purposes. With time many of them have emerged as effective herbal remedies against acute and chronic diseases. Culinary, recreational, and medicinal uses of spices and herbs has triggered vigorous scientific research in the last decades, and their antioxidant, anti-inflammatory, anticancer, anti-infectious, and glucose- and cholesterol-lowering activities were extensively studied. Many of them were also found to be effective in the prevention of neurological disorders and age related diseases. Research on various aspects of the science of spices over the past decades has established interesting linkages between their taste and olfactory properties and the bioactive constituents that they possess. These include sulfur-containing compounds, tannins, alkaloids, steroids, phenolic diterpenes, vitamins, flavonoids, and polyphenols.

Interestingly no "all-inclusive spices and culinary herbs list" exists. Every region of the world has its own set of spices as part of their cultural heritage and culinary practices. Research and development in the field of spices and herbs are the focus of this new book series entitled, *"Science of Spices and Culinary Herbs"*. The 1st volume of the book series was well received. The present 2nd volume of this book series has 6 reviews, written by leading experts and covers various aspects of the science of spices. These articles focus on 6 common spices and culinary herbs with reference to their ethnomedicinal, nutritional and culinary properties, whereas their therapeutics and biological properties are cross cutting themes in these chapters.

Tamarind (*Tamarindus indica* L.) is among the most famous spices and a culinary herb. It is an essential ingredient of many summer drinks in the South Asian region. The review by Kakudidi *et al.* provides an excellent overview of the ethnomedicinal uses, conservation work, and pre-clinical and clinical studies conducted on Tamarind. Black pepper (*Piper nigrum* L.) is the focus of the article contributed by Pimple *et al*. They discuss its traditional uses, phytochemistry, and pharmacology, as well as recent research on its beneficial role in the management of diabetes, obesity and cardiovascular diseases. Bashir and Safdar have reviewed recent work on a famous sub-continental herb, Coriander (*Coriandrum sativum* L.) including its ethnomedicinal and culinary uses. Its antioxidant, antidiabetic, cholesterol lowering, anti-inflammatory, hepatoprotective and anticancer properties are also discussed. Maan *et al.* have contributed a comprehensive review on the phytochemistry and pharmacology of Fenugreek (*Trigonella foenum-graecum* L.), particularly on the numerous pre-clinical and clinical studies conducted due to its antidiabetic properties. Anitha Rajasekaran's article is based on traditional and modern uses of famous herb Fennel (*Foeniculum vulgare* Mill.), including its major constituents and various pharmacological properties. The last chapter of the volume is on Dill seed (*Anethum graveolens* L.), contributed by More *et al.* They have reviewed the therapeutic potential of Dill seed constituents and their mechanism of action at the molecular level.

All the authors of this volume deserve our appreciation for their excellent scholarly contributions, and for the timely submissions of their review articles. The production team of Bentham Science Publishers also deserves our appreciation for a job well done. Among them Ms. Fariya Zulfiqar (Manager Publications), and Mr. Mahmood Alam (Director Publications) of Bentham Science Publishers have played a key role in the timely completion of the volume in hand. We sincerely hope that the efforts of the authors and the production team will help readers in getting a better understanding of the therapeutic benefits of colourful and aromatic spices and herbs, which we enjoy every day in our cuisines and in our salad bowls.

Atta-ur-Rahman *FRS*
Kings College, University of Cambridge
Cambridge
UK

M. Iqbal Choudhary, & Sammer Yousuf
H.E.J. Research Institute of Chemistry
International Center for Chemical and Biological Sciences
University of Karachi
Karachi
Pakistan

List of Contributors

Abid A. Maan	National Institute of Food Science and Technology, University of Agriculture, Faisalabad, Pakistan
Amrita M. Kulkarni	P. E. Society's Modern College of Pharmacy, Yamunanagar, Nigdi, Pune, India
Anitha Rajasekaran	Department of Botany, Bharathi Women's college, Prakasam Salai, Broadway, Chennai-600108, India
Asif Safdar	Department of Pharmacy, Capital University of Science and Technology, Islamabad, Pakistan
Bhushan P. Pimple	P. E. Society's Modern College of Pharmacy, Yamunanagar, Nigdi, Pune, India
Esezah K. Kakudidi	Department of Plant Sciences, Microbiology & Biotechnology, College of Natural Sciences, Makerere University, P.O. Box 7062 Kampala, Uganda
Farhan Zameer	School of Basic and Applied Science, Department of Biological Sciences, Dayananda Sagar University, Shavige Malleshwara Hills, Kumaraswamy Layout, Bengaluru - 560 078, Karnataka, India
Godwin Anywar	Department of Plant Sciences, Microbiology & Biotechnology, College of Natural Sciences, Makerere University, P.O. Box 7062 Kampala, Uganda
Govindappa Melappa	Department of Biotechnology, Dayananda Sagar College of Engineering, Dayananda Sagar Institutions, Shavige Malleshwara Hills, Kumaraswamy Layout, Bengaluru - 560 078, Karnataka, India
Kounaina Khan	Department of Dravyaguna, JSS Ayurvedic Medical College, Lalithadripura, Mysuru - 570 028, Karnataka, India
Muhammad A. Hafeez	National Institute of Food Science and Technology, University of Agriculture, Faisalabad, Pakistan
Pankaj Satapathy	School of Basic and Applied Science, Department of Biological Sciences, Dayananda Sagar University, Shavige Malleshwara Hills, Kumaraswamy Layout, Bengaluru - 560 078, Karnataka, India
Patience Tugume	Department of Plant Sciences, Microbiology & Biotechnology, College of Natural Sciences, Makerere University, P.O. Box 7062 Kampala, Uganda
Ruchita B. Bhor	P. E. Society's Modern College of Pharmacy, Yamunanagar, Nigdi, Pune, India
Samuel Ojelel	Department of Plant Sciences, Microbiology & Biotechnology, College of Natural Sciences, Makerere University, P.O. Box 7062 Kampala, Uganda
Samra Bashir	Department of Pharmacy, Capital University of Science and Technology, Islamabad, Pakistan
Sana Riaz	National Institute of Food Science and Technology, University of Agriculture, Faisalabad, Pakistan
S. Aishwarya	School of Basic and Applied Science, Department of Biological Sciences, Dayananda Sagar University, Shavige Malleshwara Hills, Kumaraswamy Layout, Bengaluru - 560 078, Karnataka, India
Shivaprasad Hudeda	Department of Dravyaguna, JSS Ayurvedic Medical College, Lalithadripura, Mysuru - 570 028, Karnataka, India

Sunil S. More   School of Basic and Applied Science, Department of Biological Sciences, Dayananda Sagar University, Shavige Malleshwara Hills, Kumaraswamy Layout, Bengaluru - 560 078, Karnataka, India

Veena SM   Department of Biotechnology, Sapthagiri Engineering College, Bangalore, India

Tamarind (*Tamarindus indica* L.): A Review of its Use as a Spice, a Culinary Herb and Medicinal Applications

Patience Tugume, Godwin Anywar, Samuel Ojelel and **Esezah K. Kakudidi**

Department of Plant Sciences, Microbiology & Biotechnology, College of Natural Sciences, Makerere University, P.O. Box 7062 Kampala, Uganda

Abstract: Tamarind (*Tamarindus indica*) is a highly valued multipurpose fruit tree indigenous to tropical Africa. *T. indica* is extensively used in traditional medicine and has been widely studied. Different authors have provided reviews on the various aspects of tamarind, with a focus on its traditional uses, ecology, phytochemistry and pharmacology. Limited studies on the preclinical and clinical aspects of tamarind have been explored in most reviews. Even less attention has been given to the use of tamarind as a spice or a culinary herb. This chapter reviews the health benefits of tamarind as a spice and a culinary herb. It also explores the choice of tamarind use over other spices and how it is utilized to improve people's livelihoods. The ethnomedicinal uses of tamarind are supported with recent scientific evidence from preclinical and clinical studies. The threats to the sustainable use of tamarind, particularly environmental degradation, land conversion and climate change are discussed. We conclude by highlighting the conservation strategies that are currently being implemented to ensure sustainable utilization of tamarind.

Keywords: Conservation, Culinary herb, Economic potential, Ethnomedicinal, Preclinical and clinical, Spice, *Tamarindus indica*.

INTRODUCTION

Tamarind (*Tamarindus indica* L.) is a monotypic genus of the family Fabaceae. The species is known by various local names in different parts of the world [1 - 3]. Geographically, tamarind grows in 54 countries and is indigenous to 18 tropical African countries. Its range runs along the dryland zone from Senegal in the west through Sudan and Ethiopia in the east, extending southward to Mozambique and Madagascar [4]. It is introduced in 36 other countries where it is cultivated in subtropical Asia but naturalized in Spain, North and South America

* **Corresponding Author Esezah K. Kakudidi:** Department of Plant Sciences, Microbiology & Biotechnology, College of Natural Sciences, Makerere University, P.O. Box 7062 Kampala, Uganda; Tel: +256 712 929254; E-mail esezahk@gmail.com

Atta-ur-Rahman, M. Iqbal Choudhary & Sammer Yousuf

[2, 5, 6]. The use of tamarind in traditional medicine and food processing has been widely studied [5, 7 - 9]. Different authors have carried out reviews on the various aspects of tamarind, with a focus on its traditional uses, ecology, phytochemistry and pharmacology [10 - 12]. Limited studies on preclinical and clinical aspects of tamarind have been explored in reviews [3, 11].

Tamarind has been exploited to improve people's livelihoods [5, 13 - 15]. Much of the tamarind is extracted from the wild and this poses a threat to its sustainable use [15], although there are exceptions where it is grown in plantations [5]. This chapter explores the scientific evidence from preclinical and clinical studies of the health benefits of tamarind, its use as a spice and medicine. It also emphasizes other uses of tamarind and its conservation strategies.

OBJECTIVES

The main objective of this chapter is to combine the recent developments and evidence supporting the use of *T. indica* as a spice and a medicine from the preclinical and clinical perspectives. In addition, the chapter highlights the contribution of *T. indica* to livelihood improvement and the strategies towards its conservation.

METHODS

Information was gathered from published sources including scholarly journal articles, books, reports and conference proceedings. The search engines and databases used included Web of Science, Research4Life, PubMed, Google scholar, and ScienceDirect. '*Tamarindus indica*' was the key word for English language searches only in combination with other relevant terms. The searches were then refined to look out for specific information pertaining to the uses of *T. indica* as a spice, culinary herb, medicine and other uses. The search also emphasized preclinical and clinical trials of the various parts of tamarind used in traditional medicine.

TAMARIND AS A CULINARY HERB AND SPICE

A spice is a seed, fruit, root, bark, or other plant substances primarily used for flavouring, colouring or preserving food. Culinary herbs are the leaves, flowers, or stems of plants used for flavouring or as a garnish [16, 17].

Tamarind is a multipurpose tropical tree that has found worldwide applications. It is valued especially for its fruit, which is widely eaten fresh or processed as a seasoning or spice [18]. As such there are ethnic variations in the knowledge, value of its use and preparation of tamarind products [19] possibly due to 'ethnobotanic drift' where the parts used were originally selected by chance [4, 7, 10, 13]; or through interaction with other cultures [20]. For instance, in West Africa Van der Stege *et al.* [7] reported 250 different ways of tamarind use categorized as medicinal, nutritional, spiritual, ethnoveterinary and other uses while Ashfaque *et al.* [3] emphasized its use in traditional Unani medicine in Asia. A range of processed products from tamarind are made by utilizing its pods, leaves, seeds, seedlings, flowers, and fruit pulp [5, 12, 14].

Leaves, Flowers and Seedlings

The tender leaves, flowers and seedlings of *T. indica* are cooked and eaten as vegetables [21]. The leaves are available throughout the year and can be used when green or dried [7] to provide alternative curries in many countries, although in other parts of the world, the leaves are consumed as a famine food [10]. However, removal of leaves affects fruit production and yield [10], and therefore, their harvesting should be done cautiously. Since African diets are generally poor in micronutrients, the leaves add vitamins and minerals to the staple starchy crop-based diets for many rural people. The flowers of tamarind are also used in traditional food preparations in West Africa [7].

Fruits and Pulp

The tender raw tamarind pods are used to prepare pickles [12, 22]. The immature pods are boiled with porridge to give it a sour taste in Uganda [13]. In India, they are used for seasoning rice, meat, fish and other sauces. They are also salted and eaten, while the unripe mature fruits are roasted in coal and dipped in wood ash before being eaten in the Bahamas [23].

The mature ripe fruits are harvested when the pulp is brownish-red. The fruit pulp is the major part used in traditional dishes, drinks, and seasoning as a spice processed through different pathways [7]. The fruit pulp may be eaten as a snack or processed into juice or fermented into wine [24]. It can also be processed into jams and sweets or used as a raw material in the manufacture of several industrial products: flavouring confections, curries and sauces, concentrates, pulp powder, tartaric acid, pectin, tartarates and alcohol [5, 10, 20, 23]. In East Africa, tamarind pulp is cooked with maize meal and made into porridge called Ugali. In Eastern Uganda, the tamarind fruit is used as food, beverage, a spice and a preservative. The pulp is also used to enhance the taste and flavour of meat, and to improve the consistency of boiled potatoes [13].

Seeds

The seeds are an abundant by-product of the tamarind pulp industry [25]. The presence of tannins and other dying materials in the seed testa makes it unfit for direct consumption [10]. However, the seeds can be consumed after removal of the testa by soaking and boiling in water or roasting. The cotyledons are ground into flour which may be made into cakes or bread [5]. The roasted seeds are claimed to be superior to groundnuts in flavour [2, 14]. In Ghana and India, the seeds are pounded and eaten in times of famine [5, 26]. The seeds contain about 46-48% jellose which is important in fruit preservation [5]. The kennel powder is also used in the confectionary industry and as a stabilizer in ice cream, mayonnaise and cheese [5, 27].

Choice of Tamarind over Other Spices

Spices are the building blocks of flavours and set apart one cuisine from another. They define the flavours and cuisines, and are important elements for providing consistency or colour. Today's consumers are becoming sophisticated about the choices and use of spices [17]. The choice of spices depends on regional preferences, cooking style, distinct flavour and properties, dietary beliefs, culture, and ecological availability that are linked to environmental concerns and health benefits [17]. *T. indica* exhibits a wide range of physiological properties that enhance taste, flavour, aroma, texture, and colour/visual appeal, its application in food preservation and as a digestive stimulant [28, 29].

The most outstanding characteristic of tamarind is its sweet acidic taste, due to the presence of tartaric acid ranging from 12.2-23.8%, which is uncommon in other plant tissues [23]. Although tartaric acid occurs in other sour fruits, such as grapes, grapefruits and raspberries, it is not present in such high proportions as in tamarind. The sourness and aroma of young leaves make them ideal as seasoning vegetables [30]. In the absence of tamarind pulp, the leaves are preferred over other sour fruits since fewer leaves are needed to obtain the required acidic taste.

Jellose from tamarind seeds is a good food gelling and stabilizing agent [25]. Gelling is a superior preservation technique for fruits. In comparison to other natural gelling fruit/seed substances, tamarind forms gel at low water activity, that is, at sugar concentration >60%. Therefore, jellose is a good choice when considering the versatile products in which it can be added as a stabilizer: ice cream, mayonnaise and cheese, jam, jellies and marmalades. It also improves the viscosity and texture of processed foods; crispness and thickness of biscuits [25].

Tamarind has abundant volatile compounds such as 2-acetyl-furan and 5-methylfurfural which form its aroma. Additionally, 2-phenyl acetaldehyde imparts the fruity and honey-like odour; 2- furfuryl, a caramel-like flavour while hexadecenoic acid and limonene impart a citrus flavour [31 - 33]. The preference of tamarind as a food colourant is attributed to leucoanthocyanidin and anthocyanin pigments which give the red colour [34, 35]. In comparison to other spices like chili pepper, garlic, 'Pak kyheng' (Thai leafy vegetable), shallot and turmeric, tamarind enhances iron availability and absorption in the intestines [34]. The use of tamarind is thus helpful in the prevention and treatment of anaemia in children and pregnant mothers, whose iron demand is often high [36]. The high risk of constipation-related haemorrhoids and hypotension often encountered in anaemic pregnant women with iron supplementation could be counteracted since tamarind is a laxative.

HEALTH AND OTHER BENEFITS OF TAMARIND

Plants are the basic components in traditional medicine with over 80% of the world's population especially in developing countries depending on them [37, 38]. All parts of *T. indica* are used in traditional medicine [12, 20, 22]. However, there are cultural, ethnic and or regional differences in methods of preparation and administration [3, 4, 12, 22].

The different parts of *T. indica* are reported to improve one's overall health if consumed on a regular basis as they have rich nutritional and calorific value [5, 11]. *T. indica* is used traditionally to treat abdominal pain, diarrhoea and dysentery, helminths infections, wounds, malaria and fever, constipation, inflammation, snake and scorpion bites, gonorrhoea, eye diseases and plant poisoning [10, 20, 22, 39]. The scope of traditional medicine use has been extensively reviewed in Africa [4, 40], Unani [3] and Ayuverdic medicine [12].

T. indica contains many chemical compounds as extensively discussed in various reports [10, 25, 41, 42]. The leaves and flowers contain proteins, vitamin C, beta-carotene and a high content of potassium, phosphorus, calcium and magnesium [23].

PHYTOMEDICINE SUPPORTED WITH PRE-CLINICAL STUDIES

Tamarind has been subjected to extensive phytochemical, experimental and clinical investigations that have demonstrated its analgesic, anthelmintic, antiasthmatic, antiatherosclerosis, antidiabetic, anti-emetic, antiinflammatory, antimicrobial, anti-nociceptive, antioxidant, antiulcer, fungicidal, hepato-protective, nephroprotective, hypolipidemic, anti-venom, immunomodulatory effects, and antiathritic [3, 43 - 48]. Scientific studies have confirmed different traditional claims of the medicinal benefits of *T. indica* [4, 49]. Some of the scientifically validated claims of the different parts of *T. indica* are highlighted in the following preclinical studies.

Anthelmintic

The juice of *T. indica* leaves showed significant antihelmintic activity when compared with the standard antihelmintic drug Piperazine citrate [50]. Hurtada *et al.* [51] demonstrated the effectiveness of *T. indica* leaves decoction against gastrointestinal nematodes of goats namely: *Trichostrongylus* spp., *Oesophagostomum* spp., *Haemonchus* spp. and *Bunostomum* spp.

A study to determine the mortality of *Ascaris suum* exposed to different concentrations of *T. indica* seed extract showed that it was potent after 12 hours at 80% concentration [52]. Tamarind seeds possess significant anthelmintic activities and are a potential alternative for management of helminths to solve chemical resistance and economic problems in small farms [52].

Anti-asthmatic

The methanolic extract of *T. indica* leaves exhibited significant antihistaminic, adaptogenic and mast cell stabilizing activity in laboratory animals [53]. The anti-inflammatory activity of *T. indica* pulp extract improved breathing patterns in animal models of asthma that had been induced with histamine dihydrochloride [54].

Antibacterial

Extracts from *T. indica* flowers are highly active against *Staphylococcus aureus* with low Minimum Inhibitory Concentration (MIC) values of 25 µg/ml [55]. Polyphenols and flavonoids in leaf extracts of *T. indica* are responsible for the antibacterial activity against *S. aureus* and *Pseudomonas aeruginosa* [56]. The leaf extracts also possess a strong *in vitro* antibacterial activity against more than 13 common gram positive and gram-negative bacteria [57].

An aqueous fruit pulp extract showed antibacterial activity against *S. aureus*, *Escheriachia coli* and *P. aeruginosa* with the exception of *Salmonella typhii* [58]. Crude ethanol extracts of *T. indica* showed strong antibacterial activity against *E. coli*, *Klebsiella pneumonia*, *Salmonella paratyphi* A and *P. aeruginosa* [59]. These microorganisms are aetiological agents in urinary tract infections (UTI), wounds, pneumonia and paratyphoid fever. Daniyan & Muhammad [59] noted that *P. aeruginosa* is resistant to a majority of antibiotics and therefore this response to *T. indica* extracts warrants further *in vivo* and clinical investigations after isolation and characterization of the bioactive components.

With the exception of *Bacillus subtilis*, the aqueous and ethanol extracts of *T. indica* leaves showed poor or no antibacterial and antifungal activity against

Enterococcus faecalis, *S. aureus*, *E. coli*, *Salmonella typhimurium*, *P. aeruginosa* and *Candida albicans*. However, the pure essential oils from the leaves showed a broad antibacterial spectrum [41]. The bark extract of *T. indica* also showed antimicrobial activity against *S. pneumoniae*, *E. coli* and *S. paratyphi* [60].

Wound Healing

T. indica fruit extracts showed wound healing effects by significantly reducing the healing time in mice [61]. Delayed wound healing is often associated with the presence of a number of microorganisms such as *P. aeruginosa*, *S. aureus*, *S. faecalis*, *E. coli*, *Clostridium perfringens*, *C. tetani*, *Coliform bacilli* and *Enterococcus* [62]. The presence of tannins in *T. indica* fruit pulp could therefore be associated with faster wound healing due to its antimicrobial property.

Hypoglycaemic

The stem-bark extract of *T. indica* was investigated for its hypoglycaemic action on experimentally induced hyperglycaemic Wistar rats using a single dose of alloxan monohydrate (150 mg/kg, IP). It significantly lowered the elevated blood glucose level (BGL), and prevented an elevation in BGL when used in the oral glucose load model [63]. A study by Agnihotri & Singh [64] showed a significant decrease in BGL in diabetic rats, treated with the alcohol extracts of the stem bark of *T. indica*.

Tamarind seeds also lowered blood glucose and enhanced storage of glycogen in Sprague Dawley rats [65]. The hydroethanolic seed coat extract of *T. indica* exhibited potent hypoglycaemic action in alloxan induced rats [20].

Antioxidant

The alcohol extract of stem bark of *T. indica* showed significant antioxidant activity [60] with no signs of toxicity up to of 2000 mg/p.o in acute toxicity studies [64, 66]. Vasant and Narasimhacharya [67] also demonstrated the therapeutic effects of *T. indica* leaf as an antioxidant as well as having antihyperglycaemic, antihyperlipidaemic and antiperoxidative properties.

Anti-inflammatory

T. indica seed extract had significant anti-inflammatory activity on nitric oxide (NO) and tumour necrosis factor-α (TNF-α). Additionally, it exhibited a favourable effect on β-cell neogenesis and improved mRNA concentration of sterol regulatory element-binding proteins (SREBP-1c) [68]. Orally administered hydroethanolic extracts of *T. indica* leaves showed significant dose-dependent anti-inflammatory and antinociceptive properties in male Wister albino rats [20].

Antiviral

T. indica stem bark extracts showed antiviral activity against Newcastle Disease. It has been recommended as a potential antiviral drug [69].

Chemoprotective

T. indica showed chemoprotective activity against the development of colon cancer in hypercholesterolemic hamsters, which were exposed to the carcinogen dimethylhydrazine (DMH) [66]. The chemoprotective activity also has the potential of lowering the risk of atherosclerosis.

Antinociceptive/ Analgesic

The aqueous fruit extract of *T. indica* exerted a significant peripheral and central analgesic effects in rodent models probably due to the activation of the opioidergic mechanism [70], and therefore a potential for reducing pain. The methanolic extract of *T. indica* seeds produced a significant reduction in pain and inflammation demonstrating analgesic and anti-inflammatory activity *in vivo* in Wistar albino rats [69, 70].

Hypolipidemic & Hypotensive

The ethanolic extract of *T. indica* fruit pulp also showed significant weight reduction and hypolipidemic activity in cafeteria diet and sulpiride-induced obese rats [71]. The seeds of *T. indica* also lowered serum cholesterol levels in Sprague Dawley rats [65].

Anti-fungal

The aqueous and ethanolic fruit pulp extracts of *T. indica* were effective against *C. albicans* at 475 and 485 mg/ml respectively, which doubled as the Minimum Inhibitory and Minimum Fungicidal Concentration (MIC and MFC) in both extracts [72].

Aphrodisiac

T. indica pulp showed aphrodisiac and spermatogenic activity in male Wistar rats [73]. There was a significant improvement in sexual desire (mount and intromission frequency) and parameters of sexual arousal comparable to the standard drug sildenafil citrate. There was a significant increase in sperm production and motility without any sign of toxicity in testis from histopathological examination.

Peptic Ulcer

The *T. indica* seed extract showed a dose dependent protective effect on animal peptic ulcer models induced by ibuprofen, alcohol and pyrolus ligation [74]. *T. indica* leaf extract was also found to have anti-ulcerogenic and ulcer healing properties in rats, which might also be due to its anti-secretory and antioxidant properties [75].

Nephroprotective

T. indica seed extracts ameliorated chemically induced nephrotoxicity and renal cell carcinoma in animal models [76].

Hepatoprotective

Supplementation of rat diet with tamarind seed extract (TSE) significantly inhibited oxidative burst in the liver and maintained homeostasis. This demonstrated the protective efficacy of TSE against arthritis-associated oxidative liver damage [47]. A study to evaluate the protective effect of *T. indica* fruit pulp extract on the collagen content and oxidative stress in liver and kidney of fluoride-exposed rats showed that supplementation with tamarind alleviated the adverse effects of fluoride [77].

Anti-Snake-Venom

T. indica seed extract inhibited the enzymatic effects induced by *Vipera russelli* venom in a dose-dependent manner. Thus, the seed extract could be used as an alternative treatment to serum therapy [78].

Antiarthritic

Septic arthritis generally requires a long-term treatment by antibiotics. In comparison, the ethanolic extract of *T. indica* leaves was effective against septic arthritis caused by *S. aureus* in rabbits when administered orally at 1000 mg/kg for 14 consecutive days. This is a potential alternative for the treatment of septic arthritis in human beings [79]. The aqueous and alcohol extracts of *T. indica* seed coat also significantly inhibited paw oedema-induced arthritis in rats. The alcohol extract activity was higher than the standard drugs and untreated control. *T. indica* has anti-inflammatory, antinociceptive, and antiarthritic effects in arthritic rats [48]. Additionally, *T. indica* seed extract exhibited cartilage and bone protection by inhibiting the activities of degradative enzymes. It also mitigated the augmented levels of inflammatory mediators and alleviated increased levels of reactive oxygen species [47].

Ameliorative Effects of *T. indica* in Fluoride Poisoning

Fluoride poisoning is a health hazard that damages the carbohydrate, lipid and antioxidant metabolisms. Fluorosis has limited remedial measures. Administration of *T. indica* leaf extract to albino rats exposed to fluoride poisoning simulating diabetic and hyperlipidaemic conditions restored carbohydrate, lipid and antioxidant metabolism [67]. Gupta *et al.* [80] also demonstrated the ameliorative effects of *T. indica* fruit pulp on fluoride poisoning *via* the down regulation of type 1 collagen mRNA in dentin of incisor teeth of rats. *T. indica* fruit pulp supplementation increased urinary excretion of fluoride while decreasing the retention of fluoride in bone [81]. Accordingly, Khandare *et al.* [81], correlated daily consumption of tamarind with less dental and skeletal fluorosis.

Immunomodulatory

Galactoxyloglucan (PST001), isolated from seed kernel of *T. indica* is a non-toxic immunostimulatory agent [82]. *T. indica* seeds contain a polysaccharide with immunomodulatory properties such as phagocytic enhancement; leucocyte migration and cell proliferation inhibition. The seed kernel of *T. indica* caused an increase in total WBC, CD4+ T-cell population, and bone marrow cellularity, suggestive of a potent immunomodulatory activity [83 - 85].

Anticancer/Antitumor

The evaluation of the antitumour activity of galactoxyloglucan polysaccharide, (PST001) isolated from the seed kernel of *T. indica* showed significant tumour reduction in the murine cancer cell lines DLA and EAC. Thus, PST001 is a potential anticancer agent [82, 83].

A combination of PST001 and nanoparticles of doxorubicin, a commonly used drug to treat human malignancies showed superior therapeutic efficiency while retaining the cytotoxic effects of PST001 even at lower concentrations. PST-Dox combination is selectively cytotoxic against cancer cells through the induction of apoptosis *in vitro* [86]. PST001 has the potential of being developed as an anticancer agent that not only preserves innate biological activity of tumour necrosis factor-related apoptosis-inducing ligand (TRAIL), but also sensitizes cancer cells to TRAIL-mediated apoptosis [85, 87, 88].

Safety/Toxicity

There is little information available on the safety and or toxicity of *T. indica*. Silva *et al.* [89] evaluated the clastogenic and/or genotoxic potential of *T. indica* fruit pulp extract *in vivo* in peripheral blood and liver cells of Wistar rats and in bone marrow cells of Swiss mice at doses of 1000, 1500 and 2000 mg/kg body weight. In addition, Silva *et al*. [89] concluded that *T. indica* fruit pulp extract did not induce clastogenic/ aneugenic or cytotoxic effects on liver enzymes or DNA damage. Martinello *et al*. [43] indicated that the higher concentrations of *T. indica* extract administered to rats were still safe compared to the 5% concentration usually present in juice consumed by humans [43].

On the flipside, the bioassay-guided fractionation of the methanolic extract of *T. indica* fruits led to the isolation of L-(-)-di-/n-butyl malate which exhibited a pronounced cytotoxic activity against sea urchin embryo cells by inhibiting the development of the fertilized eggs [90]. The fact that the isolated compound from *T. indica* fruit pulp prevented urchin embryo development underscores the synergism of the compounds in the whole *T. indica* extracts.

CLINICAL ASPECTS OF TAMARIND

Clinical trials of any medicine require the use of standardized products. Consequently, *T. indica* has been subjected to only a few of clinical trials despite its numerous health benefits. The seeds of *T. indica* contain Xyloglucan which forms a protective biofilm on the intestinal mucus layer against chemical or bacterial aggression. Xyloglucan capsules and powders have been formulated for adults and children respectively for controlling and reducing symptoms of diarrhoea and for restoration of the physiological function of the intestinal wall in Europe [91, 92].

In a randomized clinical trial involving 150 patients in Romania, Xyloglucan proved an effective option for the treatment of acute diarrhoea as compared to two widely used antidiarrheal products: *Saccharomyces boulardii* containing the yeast probiotic, *S. boulardii* and diosmectite, an absorbent activated natural aluminosilicate clay. In another randomized clinical trial in Romania, Xyloglucan plus Oral Rehydration Salts (ORS) were more effective against acute gastroenteritis in children aged from 3 months to 12 years compared to ORS alone, thus a safe option for diarrhoeal treatment [93].

Furthermore, a herbal formulation consisting of the ethanol/aqueous extracts of *T. indica* seeds and ethanol extract of *Curcuma longa* rhizome provided significant relief from knee pain after physical activity and improved joint function in non-arthritic adults in a randomized, double-blind, placebo-controlled study [94].

The dried and pulverized pulp of *T. indica* fruits significantly lowered total cholesterol level, Low Density Lipoprotein (LDL)-cholesterol level, diastolic pressure at a dose of 15 mg/kg body weight in a randomized clinical trial [95].

OTHER USES OF *T. INDICA*

Apart from the use of different parts of the tamarind tree as a spice, a culinary herb and for medicinal purposes, it is also used for several other purposes (Table 1).

Table 1. Other uses of tamarind.

Plant Part	Use
Seed testa/ husk	Dyeing and tanning, food preservative [23].
Seed	Filler for adhesives in plywood industry, stabilizer for bricks, binder for sawdust briquettes and thickener for some explosives [5].
	Livestock feed rations [96].
	Education and learning aids during arithmetic lessons for beginners [13].
	Aesthetic use in traditional board games (mweso) [13].
Seed (Kennel) powder	Sizing material in textile, paper and jute industry [5, 97]
	Gelling, thickening and bulking agent, emulsifier, crystallisation inhibitor, preservative, improves palatability, water retainer, cold insulator and glazing agent in the food industry textile, paper and jute industry [98]
	Coagulant in water treatment, excipient in making greaseless ointment, gelatinizing agent, emulsifying agents for insecticides preparation, stabilizer in capsule formulation in the pharmaceutical industry, dentures and solution for contact lenses, thickener in explosives [98]
	Cosmetics, book binding and plywood manufacture [27]
	Xyloglucans used to improve mechanical properties of paper sheets [99].
	Oil for making paints and vanishes, burning in lamps [19, 100, 101].
	Fish poison [5].
Fruit pulp	Mixed with sea salt to polish brass, copper and silver [102, 103].
	Manufacture of tamarind fruit concentrate, tamarind powder, tartarates and alcohol [40].
	To treat trypanosomiasis in domestic animals [104].
Flowers	Honey production [23].
	Tannins as mordants in dyeing of wool, silk [23].
Pod shells	Absorbent for removal of methylene blue and amaranth dyes from aqueous solutions [105].
Leaves	Silkworm rearing [23, 106].
	Mixed with gum of figs to make chewing gum [5].
	Dyeing cloth [23].
	Mulching [13].
	Tannins for removing hair from animal hides [14].

(Table 1) cont.....

Plant Part	Use
Tree	Shade, ornamental and Agroforestry to minimize the risk of crop failure, windbreak, boundary and barrier support [19, 23, 96].
Branches	Fodder [107].
Wood	Furniture: wheels, mallets, mortars, pestles, canoes, agricultural tools [14, 19].
	Fuelwood [13].
	Gunpowder [108].
	Timber for building and wood flooring [13].

ECONOMIC POTENTIAL OF *T. INDICA*

T. indica has a wide range of domestic and industrial uses but remains an under exploited wild tree [5, 9, 10, 109]. However, the untapped potential of *T. indica* has generated research interests in value addition in India, Thailand and the Philippines [18, 110], and some African countries [9, 111, 112].

The sale of *T. indica* and its processed products boosts incomes of communities and generates foreign exchange [5]. For instance, Singh *et al* [5] reported that India exported over 10,000 tonnes of processed tamarind pulp to USA earning 100 million rupees annually. Khalid *et al*. [15] reported that Sudan exported 388.2 metric tonnes and earned USD 60,400. In Uganda much as the collection of *T. indica* fruits by rural households' accounts for 74% of their annual revenue [113], it is still minimal to meet their household requirements. In west Timor, during periods of food scarcity, tamarind fruits are processed for their pulp as an income supplement, sustaining thousands of poor families [114]. The Nature Based Enterprises (NBE) in *T. indica* products create employment opportunities for the actors involved in the value chain [8] thereby contributing to attainment of Sustainable Development Goal (SDG) 1 on eradicating poverty. In some countries little value has been added to *T. indica* and thus low reported earnings [115]. Additionally, the value of *T. indica* is not often captured in monetary terms in national accounting systems despite its wide subsistence usage [23].

In order to harness the economic potential of *T. indica*, there is need to develop capacity in propagation, value addition, commercialization and promotion of NBE [5, 111]. The *T. indica* NBE support biodiversity conservation and enhance community resilience to social and environmental threats such as climate change. It is envisaged that NBE will have a potential to contribute towards better nutrition, health, access to education creation of saving and investment opportunities thereby reducing vulnerability to financial shocks.

CONSERVATION OF *T. INDICA*

The global conservation status of *T. indica* is Least Concern (LC) [116]. However, in Uganda, Kenya, Senegal and Nigeria, it is considered of high conservation priority [112]. The species is threatened by deforestation, urbanisation, industrialization and agricultural expansion [23]. It is also harvested for timber, domestic wood fuel and for firing limestone kilns in Eastern Uganda since it produces intense heat [13].

T. indica are either self-propagating or deliberately planted. In Eastern Uganda, 52% and 45% of the *T. indica* population was self-propagated and planted respectively [13]. The trees are commonly found in wild lands and farmlands, school and administration centres' compounds. However, there is limited availability of seedlings for planting in the rural areas [13] thus limiting the expansion of its acreage.

Given that most of the *T. indica* products are extracted from wild trees, the need for conservation is paramount in order to guarantee its availability for posterity. The following are the strategies employed in the conservation for *T. indica*.

SOCIO-CULTURAL PRACTICES

T. indica is a highly sacred and worshipped tree especially in Asia. For example, some communities in India consider the tamarind tree to be haunted by spirits and is thus worshipped. In Myanmar, some communities protect the tamarind tree with a belief that they are dwelling places of their rain gods [23]. However, in Eastern Uganda, some superstitions are detrimental to planting of tamarinds such as the belief that those who plant them die without eating their fruits [13].

Plantations

The tamarind tree is easy to cultivate, free of any serious pests and diseases, and has a long life span of 150-200 years but takes 6-12 years to yield fruits [14, 18, 109]. The trees also respond to coppicing and pollarding. When establishing a pure plantation, it is recommended that spacing should be at least 13 x 13 m [14]. *T. indica* is cultivated in Asian countries with India being the world's largest producer [5, 25].

Agroforestry

T. indica is intercropped in many agroforestry systems because of its multipurpose nature. It is either preserved on farm when opening up land or integrated with agricultural crops and livestock farming [5, 13, 23] but in Thailand intensive cropping is practiced in orchards. The *T. indica* is an important tree in home gardens in South and Southeast Asia. On farm tamarind trees provide sustainable incentives to local farmers through utilization; a motivation to conserve them [23].

Germplasm

Phenotypic plasticity has been found in several species of tropical and temperate trees for many traits [117]. There is phenotypic variability in wild *T. indica* seed size, shape and colour; pod weight and length; pulp colour and taste as well as tracked and untracked bark [19]. The effect of this variability requires characterization in order to select the most interesting phenotypes/genotypes, which possess several desired traits for breeding purposes [118].

Ex-situ conservation is the easiest, economical and socially acceptable method for conserving *T. indica*. Over 100 *ex-situ* collections of *T. indica* are maintained in botanic gardens worldwide [119]. Germplasm can be maintained for a long time in seed banks and remain viable under appropriate storage conditions. This allows phenotypically superior germplasm to be collected from different regions and multiplied through vegetative propagation [23]. An important step in the domestication process is the characterization of the local natural variation of the species.

Ornamentals

T. indica is planted as an ornamental and shade tree along avenues, roadsides, parks and river banks [13, 23]. In the United States of America, the *T. indica* is used for indoor ornamentation [120].

CONCLUSION

All the parts of *T. indica* are useful with multiple local and industrial applications. As a spice and a culinary herb it offers many health benefits in traditional medicine, which have been validated by preclinical and clinical studies. Such studies underscore the potential of the different parts of *T. indica* in the development of health supplements and drugs. Despite its versatility in health, food, industry and other uses, *T. indica* remains underutilized and undervalued in most countries. The statistics on *T. indica* trade is scanty although markets for its products are available at national and international levels. The harvesting of *T. indica* that is mostly from the wild in African countries cannot meet the growing commercial demand.

RECOMMENDATIONS

In order to continually benefit from *T. indica*, the following are recommended: (i)

There is a need to boost plantation production to ensure sustainability of *T. indica* NBE; (ii) Research to explore the genetic variability in seed size and shape, pulp colour and taste, and under researched pharmacological properties such antiviral activity ; (iii) The countries where *T. indica* is underutilized should benchmark the value chain in some of the world's leading producers such as India and Thailand with regard to knowledge exchange; and (iv) organise local and international market channels in order to capture statistics on *T. indica* production and trade that would guide policy formulation regarding its conservation.

CONSENT FOR PUBLICATION

Not applicable.

CONFLICT OF INTEREST

The authors confirm that this chapter contents have no conflict of interest.

ACKNOWLEDGEMENT

We appreciate Makerere University for availing us the facilities that enabled us to conduct the review.

REFERENCES

[1]   Katende AB, Bukenya ZR, Kakudidi EK, Lye KA. Catalogue of economically important plants in Uganda. 1998.

[2]   ICRAF. Agroforestry Tree Database *Tamarindus indica* L 2007.

[3]   Ashfaque A, Wasim A, Zeenat F, Sajid M. Therapeutic, phytochemistry and pharmacology of *Tamarindus indica*: A review. Int J Unani Integr Med 2018; 2: 14-9.

[4]   Havinga RM, Hartl A, Putscher J, Prehsler S, Buchmann C, Vogl CR. *Tamarindus indica* L. (Fabaceae): patterns of use in traditional African medicine. J Ethnopharmacol 2010; 127(3): 573-88. [http://dx.doi.org/10.1016/j.jep.2009.11.028] [PMID: 19963055]

[5]   Singh D, Wangchu L, Moond SK. Processed products of Tamarind. Nat Prod Rad 2007; 6(4): 315-21.

[6]   Jyothirmayi T, Rao GN, Rao DG. Studies on instant raw tamarind chutney powder. J Foodserv 2006; 17: 119 23. [http://dx.doi.org/10.1111/j.1745-4506.2006.00027.x]

[7]   Van der Stege C, Prehsler S, Hartl A, Vogl CR. Tamarind (*Tamarindus indica* L.) in the traditional West African diet: not just a famine food. Fruits 2011; 66: 171-85. [http://dx.doi.org/10.1051/fruits/2011025]

[8]   Chiteva R, Mayunzu O, Lukibisi M, Wachira N. Enhancing Community Livelihoods through Nature Based Enterprises: Case of Matinyani Women Group, Kitui, Kenya. Environ Ecol Res 2016; 4: 30-5. [http://dx.doi.org/10.13189/eer.2016.040105]

[9]   Adeola AA, Aworh CO. Development and sensory evaluation of an improved beverage from Nigeria's tamarind (*Tamarindus indica* L.) fruit. Afr J Food Agric Nutr Dev 2010; 10(9): 1-14. [http://dx.doi.org/10.4314/ajfand.v10i9.62888]

[10]   De Caluwé E, Halamová K, Van Damme P. *Tamarindus indica* L.: a review of traditional uses,

phytochemistry and pharmacology. Afrika Focus 2010; 23: 53-83.
[http://dx.doi.org/10.21825/af.v23i1.5039]

[11]   Kuru P. *Tamarindus indica* and its health related effects. Asian Pac J Trop Biomed 2014; 4: 676-81.
[http://dx.doi.org/10.12980/APJTB.4.2014APJTB-2014-0173]

[12]   Rao YS, Mathew KM. Tamarind.Handbook of Herbs and Spices. England: Woodhead Publishing Limited 2012; pp. 512-33.

[13]   Ebifa-Othieno E, Mugisha A, Nyeko P, Kabasa JD. Knowledge, attitudes and practices in tamarind (*Tamarindus indica* L) use and conservation in Eastern Uganda. J Ethnobiol Ethnomed 2017; 13(1): 5.
[http://dx.doi.org/10.1186/s13002-016-0133-8] [PMID: 28109300]

[14]   Orwa C. Agroforestree Database: a tree reference and selection guide, version 4.0 2009.

[15]   Khalid H, El-Kamali H, Elmanan A. Trade of Sudanese natural medicinals and their role in human and wildlife health care. Crop Newsl 2007; 10: 1-5.

[16]   Opara EI, Chohan M. Culinary herbs and spices: their bioactive properties, the contribution of polyphenols and the challenges in deducing their true health benefits. Int J Mol Sci 2014; 15(10): 19183-202.
[http://dx.doi.org/10.3390/ijms151019183] [PMID: 25340982]

[17]   Raghavan S. Handbook of spices, seasonings, and flavorings. CRC press 2006.
[http://dx.doi.org/10.1201/b13597]

[18]   Gunasena HPM, Hughes A. Tamarind: *Tamarindus indica* L. International Centre for Underutilised Crops 2000.

[19]   Fandohan B, Assogbadjo AE, Kakaï RG, *et al.* Women's traditional knowledge, use value, and the contribution of tamarind (*Tamarindus indica* L.) to rural households' cash income in Benin. Econ Bot 2010; 64: 248-59.
[http://dx.doi.org/10.1007/s12231-010-9123-2]

[20]   Bhadoriya SS, Ganeshpurkar A, Narwaria J, Rai G, Jain AP. *Tamarindus indica*: Extent of explored potential. Pharmacogn Rev 2011; 5(9): 73-81.
[http://dx.doi.org/10.4103/0973-7847.79102] [PMID: 22096321]

[21]   Glew RS, Vanderjagt DJ, Chuang LT, Huang YS, Millson M, Glew RH. Nutrient content of four edible wild plants from west Africa. Plant Foods Hum Nutr 2005; 60(4): 187-93.
[http://dx.doi.org/10.1007/s11130-005-8616-0] [PMID: 16395630]

[22]   El-Siddig K, Gunasena HPM, Prasad BA, *et al.* Tamarind. *Tamarindus indica*. Southampt 2006; 13-27.

[23]   El-Siddig K, Gunasena HPM, Prasad BA, *et al.* Fruits for the future 1-Tamarind, *Tamarindus indica*. Southampton Centre for Underutilised Crops. 2006.

[24]   Iwu MM. Handbook of African medicinal plants. USA: CRC Press LLC 1993.

[25]   Bagul MB, Sonawane SK, Arya SS. Bioactive characteristics and optimization of tamarind seed protein hydrolysate for antioxidant-rich food formulations 3 Biotech 8:218 2018.

[26]   Shankaracharya NB. Tamarind-chemistry, technology and uses-a critical appraisal. J Food Sci Technol 1998; 35: 193-208.

[27]   Patil S J, nadagouder B S. Industrial Products from *Tamarindus indica*. Proc Nat Sym on Tamarindus indica L, Tirupathi (AP). organized by Forest Dept. of A.P. India, 151-5.

[28]   Sambaiah K, Srinivasan K. Effect of cumin, cinnamon, ginger, mustard and tamarind in induced hypercholesterolemic rats. Food/Nahrung 1991; 35: 47-51.
[http://dx.doi.org/10.1002/food.19910350112]

[29]   Craig HC, Jeyanthi R, Pelto G, Willford AC, Stoltzfus RJ. Using a cultural-ecological framework to explore dietary beliefs and practices during pregnancy and lactation among women in Adivasi

communities in the Nilgiris Biosphere Reserve, India. Ecol Food Nutr 2018; 57(3): 165-86.
[http://dx.doi.org/10.1080/03670244.2018.1445088] [PMID: 29509032]

[30]   Coronel RE. *Tamarindus indica* L Plant Resour South East Asia, Wageningen; Pudoc 1991; 298-301.

[31]   Carasek E, Pawliszyn J. Screening of tropical fruit volatile compounds using solid-phase microextraction (SPME) fibers and internally cooled SPME fiber. J Agric Food Chem 2006; 54(23): 8688-96.
[http://dx.doi.org/10.1021/jf0613942] [PMID: 17090108]

[32]   Vernon-Carter EJ, Espinosa-Paredes G, Beristain CI, Romero-Tehuitzil H. Effect of foaming agents on the stability, rheological properties, drying kinetics and flavour retention of tamarind foam-mats. Food Res Int 2001; 34: 587-98.
[http://dx.doi.org/10.1016/S0963-9969(01)00076-X]

[33]   Pino JA, Marbot R, Vazquez C. Volatile components of tamarind (*Tamarindus indica* L.) grown in Cuba. J Essent Oil Res 2004; 16: 318-20.
[http://dx.doi.org/10.1080/10412905.2004.9698731]

[34]   Tuntipopipat S, Zeder C, Siriprapa P, Charoenkiatkul S. Inhibitory effects of spices and herbs on iron availability. Int J Food Sci Nutr 2009; 60 (Suppl. 1): 43-55.
[http://dx.doi.org/10.1080/09637480802084844] [PMID: 18651292]

[35]   Kaur G, Nagpal A, Kaur B. Tamarind: date of India. Sci Tech Entrep 2006.

[36]   Camaschella C, Camaschella C. Iron-deficiency anemia. N Engl J Med 2015; 372(19): 1832-43.
[http://dx.doi.org/10.1056/NEJMra1401038] [PMID: 25946282]

[37]   Senthilkumar K, Aravindhan V, Rajendran A. Ethnobotanical survey of medicinal plants used by Malayali tribes in Yercaud hills of Eastern Ghats, India. J Nat Rem 2013; 13: 118-32.

[38]   WHO. Mental health global action programme (mhGAP): close the gap, dare to care. 2002.https://apps.who.int/iris/handle/10665/67222

[40]   National Research Council. Tamarind. In: Lost Crop. Africa Vol. III Fruits Washington, DC: The National Academies Press 2008; p. 149.

[41]   Escalona-Arranz JC, Péres-Roses R, Urdaneta-Laffita I, Camacho-Pozo MI, Rodríguez-Amado J, Licea-Jiménez I. Antimicrobial activity of extracts from *Tamarindus indica* L. leaves. Pharmacogn Mag 2010; 6(23): 242-7.
[http://dx.doi.org/10.4103/0973-1296.66944] [PMID: 20931087]

[42]   Rana M, Sharma P. Proximate and phytochemical screening of the seed and pulp of *Tamarind indica*. Faslnamah-i Giyahan-i Daruyi 2018; 6: 111-5.

[43]   Martinello F, Soares SM, Franco JJ, *et al.* Hypolipemic and antioxidant activities from *Tamarindus indica* L. pulp fruit extract in hypercholesterolemic hamsters. Food Chem Toxicol 2006; 44(6): 810-8.
[http://dx.doi.org/10.1016/j.fct.2005.10.011] [PMID: 16330140]

[44]   Muthu SE, Nandakumar S, Rao UA. The effect of methanolic extract of *Tamarindus indica* Linn. on the growth of clinical isolates of Burkholderia pseudomallei. Indian J Med Res 2005; 122(6): 525-8.
[PMID: 16518004]

[45]   Dhasade VV, Nirmal SA, Dighe NS, Pattan SR. An overview of *Tamarindus indica* Linn.: chemistry and pharmacological profile. Pharmacologyonline 2009; 3: 809-20.

[46]   Razali N, Abdul Aziz A, Lim CY, Mat Junit S. Investigation into the effects of antioxidant rich extract of *Tamarindus indica* Leaf on antioxidant enzyme activities, oxidative stress and gene expression profiles in HepG2 cells. PeerJ 2015; 3e1292
[http://dx.doi.org/10.7717/peerj.1292] [PMID: 26557426]

[47]   Sundaram MS, Hemshekhar M, Santhosh MS, *et al.* Tamarind Seed (*Tamarindus indica*) Extract Ameliorates Adjuvant-Induced Arthritis *via* Regulating the Mediators of Cartilage/Bone Degeneration, Inflammation and Oxidative Stress. Sci Rep 2015; 5: 11117.

[http://dx.doi.org/10.1038/srep11117] [PMID: 26059174]

[48] Babaria P, Mute V, Awari D, Ghodasara J. Invivo evaluation of antiarthritic activity of seed coat of *Tamarindus indica* Linn. Int J Pharm Pharm Sci 2011; 3: 204-7.

[49] De Caluwé E, Halamová K, Van Damme P. Tamarind (*Tamarindus indica* L.): a review of traditional uses, phytochemistry and pharmacology. Afrika Focus 2010; 23(1): 53-83.

[50] Mute VM, Keta A, Patel KS, Mirchandani D, Parth C. Anthelmintic effect of *Tamarind indica* linn leaves juice extract on Pheretima posthuma. Int J pharma. Res Dev 2009; 7: 1-6.

[51] Hurtada JMUPA, Divina BP, Ducusin RJT. Anthelmintic efficacy of jackfruit (*Artocarpus heterophyllus* L.) and tamarind (*Tamarindus indica* L.) leaves decoction against gastrointestinal nematodes of goats. Philipp J Vet Anim Sci 2012; 38(2): 157-66.

[52] Nicolas AC, Acero LH. Anthelmintic Potential of Tamarind (*Tamarindus indica*). Seeds. Int J Biosci Biochem Bioinforma 2009; 9(3): 194-201.

[53] Tayade PM, Ghaisas MM, Jagtap SA, Dongre SH. Anti-asthmatic activity of methanolic extract of leaves of *Tamarindus indica* Linn. J Pharm Res 2009; 2: 944-7.

[54] Rifa'atul M, Adnyana IK, Kurnia N. Anti-Asthma Activity of Tamarind Pulp Extract (*Tamarindus indica* L.). Int J Curr Pharm Res 2017; 9: 102.
      [http://dx.doi.org/10.22159/ijcpr.2017.v9i3.19986]

[55] Al-Fatimi M, Wurster M, Schröder G, Lindequist U. Antioxidant, antimicrobial and cytotoxic activities of selected medicinal plants from Yemen. J Ethnopharmacol 2007; 111(3): 657-66.
      [http://dx.doi.org/10.1016/j.jep.2007.01.018] [PMID: 17306942]

[56] Lima ZM, da Trindade LS, Santana GC, *et al.* Effect of *Tamarindus indica* L. and Manihot esculenta extracts on antibiotic-resistant bacteria. Pharmacognosy Res 2017; 9(2): 195-9.
      [PMID: 28539745]

[57] Meléndez PA, Capriles VA. Antibacterial properties of tropical plants from Puerto Rico. Phytomedicine 2006; 13(4): 272-6.
      [http://dx.doi.org/10.1016/j.phymed.2004.11.009] [PMID: 16492531]

[58] Abukakar MG, Ukwuani AN, Shehu RA. Phytochemical screening and antibacterial activity of *Tamarindus indica* pulp extract. Asian J Biochem 2008; 3: 134-8.
      [http://dx.doi.org/10.3923/ajb.2008.134.138]

[59] Daniyan SY, Muhammad HB. Evaluation of the antimicrobial activities and phytochemical properties of extracts of *Tamaridus indica* against some diseases causing bacteria. Afr J Biotechnol 2008; 7: 2451-3.

[60] Srinivas G, Raja Kumar R. Antioxidant and antimicrobial activities of ethanol bark extract from *Tamarindus indica*. Int J Phytomedicine 2013; 5(3): 322-9.

[61] Bin Mohamad MY, Akram HB, Bero DN, Rahman MT. Tamarind Seed Extract Enhances Epidermal Wound Healing. Int J Biol 2011; 4: 81.
      [http://dx.doi.org/10.5539/ijb.v4n1p81]

[62] Bowler PG, Duerden BI, Armstrong DG. Wound microbiology and associated approaches to wound management. Clin Microbiol Rev 2001; 14(2): 244-69.
      [http://dx.doi.org/10.1128/CMR.14.2.244-269.2001] [PMID: 11292638]

[63] Yerima M, Anuka JA, Salawu OA, Abdu-Aguye I. Antihyperglycaemic activity of the stem-bark extract of *Tamarindus indica* L. on experimentally induced hyperglycaemic and normoglycaemic Wistar rats. Pak J Biol Sci 2014; 17(3): 414-8.
      [http://dx.doi.org/10.3923/pjbs.2014.414.418] [PMID: 24897797]

[64] Agnihotri A, Singh V. Effect of *Tamarindus indica* Linn. and *Cassia fistula* Linn. stem bark extracts on oxidative stress and diabetic conditions. Acta Pol Pharm 2013; 70(6): 1011-9.
      [PMID: 24383324]

[65]   Uchenna UE, Shori AB, Baba AS. *Tamarindus indica* seeds improve carbohydrate and lipid metabolism: An *in vivo* study. J Ayurveda Integr Med 2018; 9(4): 258-65.
[http://dx.doi.org/10.1016/j.jaim.2017.06.004] [PMID: 29203351]

[66]   Martinello F, Kannen V, Franco JJ, *et al.* Chemopreventive effects of a *Tamarindus indica* fruit extract against colon carcinogenesis depends on the dietary cholesterol levels in hamsters. Food Chem Toxicol 2017; 107(Pt A): 261-9.
[http://dx.doi.org/10.1016/j.fct.2017.07.005] [PMID: 28687269]

[67]   Vasant RA, Narasimhacharya AVRL. Ameliorative effect of tamarind leaf on fluoride-induced metabolic alterations. Environ Health Prev Med 2012; 17(6): 484-93.
[http://dx.doi.org/10.1007/s12199-012-0277-7] [PMID: 22438201]

[68]   Sole SS, Srinivasan BP. Aqueous extract of tamarind seeds selectively increases glucose transporter-2, glucose transporter-4, and islets' intracellular calcium levels and stimulates β-cell proliferation resulting in improved glucose homeostasis in rats with streptozotocin-induced diabetes mellitus. Nutr Res 2012; 32(8): 626-36.
[http://dx.doi.org/10.1016/j.nutres.2012.06.015] [PMID: 22935346]

[69]   Okoh OO, Obiiyeke GE, Nwodo UU, Okoh AI. Ethanol extract and chromatographic fractions of *Tamarindus indica* stem bark inhibits Newcastle disease virus replication. Pharm Biol 2017; 55(1): 1806-8.
[http://dx.doi.org/10.1080/13880209.2017.1331364] [PMID: 28539068]

[70]   Khalid S, Shaik Mossadeq WM, Israf DA, *et al. In vivo* analgesic effect of aqueous extract of *Tamarindus indica* L. fruits. Med Princ Pract 2010; 19(4): 255-9.
[http://dx.doi.org/10.1159/000312710] [PMID: 20516700]

[71]   Jindal V, Dhingra D, Sharma S, Parle M, Harna RK. Hypolipidemic and weight reducing activity of the ethanolic extract of *Tamarindus indica* fruit pulp in cafeteria diet- and sulpiride-induced obese rats. J Pharmacol Pharmacother 2011; 2(2): 80-4.
[http://dx.doi.org/10.4103/0976-500X.81896] [PMID: 21772765]

[72]   Adedayo MR, Babatunde SK, Ajiboye AE, Habeeb LM. Antimycotic and phytochemical screening of the fruit pulp extract of Tamarind (*Tamarindus indica*) on *Candida albicans.* J Microbiol Antimicrob Agents 2016; 2: 16-21.

[73]   Rai A, Das S, Chamallamudi MR, *et al.* Evaluation of the aphrodisiac potential of a chemically characterized aqueous extract of *Tamarindus indica* pulp. J Ethnopharmacol 2018; 210: 118-24.
[http://dx.doi.org/10.1016/j.jep.2017.08.016] [PMID: 28830817]

[74]   Kalra P, Sharma S, Suman SK, Kumar S. Antiulcer effect of the methanolic extract of *Tamarindus indica* seeds in different experimental models. J Pharm Bioallied Sci 2011; 3(2): 236-41.
[http://dx.doi.org/10.4103/0975-7406.80778] [PMID: 21687352]

[75]   Raja NRL, Jegan N, Wesley J. Antiulcerogenic activity of alcoholic extract of the leaves of *Tamarindus indica* (L) on experimental ulcer models. Pharmacologyonline 2008; 3: 85-92.

[76]   Vargas-Olvera CY, Sánchez-González DJ, Solano JD, *et al.* Characterization of N-diethylnitrosamin--initiated and ferric nitrilotriacetate-promoted renal cell carcinoma experimental model and effect of a tamarind seed extract against acute nephrotoxicity and carcinogenesis. Mol Cell Biochem 2012; 369(1-2): 105-17.
[http://dx.doi.org/10.1007/s11010-012-1373-0] [PMID: 22761015]

[77]   Gupta AR, Dey S, Saini M, Swarup D. Protective effect of *Tamarindus indica* fruit pulp extract on collagen content and oxidative stress induced by sodium fluoride in the liver and kidney of rats. Toxicol Environ Chem 2013; 95: 1611-23.
[http://dx.doi.org/10.1080/02772248.2014.890724]

[78]   Ushanandini S, Nagaraju S, Harish Kumar K, *et al.* The anti-snake venom properties of *Tamarindus indica* (leguminosae) seed extract. Phytother Res 2006; 20(10): 851-8.

[http://dx.doi.org/10.1002/ptr.1951] [PMID: 16847999]

[79]   Mandal P, Sinha Babu SP, Mandal NC. Antimicrobial activity of saponins from Acacia auriculiformis. Fitoterapia 2005; 76(5): 462-5.
[http://dx.doi.org/10.1016/j.fitote.2005.03.004] [PMID: 15951137]

[80]   Mohan S, Gupta D. Phytochemical analysis and differential *in vitro* cytotoxicity assessment of root extracts of *Inula racemosa*. Biomed Pharmacother 2017; 89: 781-95.
[http://dx.doi.org/10.1016/j.biopha.2017.02.053] [PMID: 28273640]

[81]   Khandare AL, Rao GS, Lakshmaiah N. Effect of tamarind ingestion on fluoride excretion in humans. Eur J Clin Nutr 2002; 56(1): 82-5.
[http://dx.doi.org/10.1038/sj.ejcn.1601287] [PMID: 11840184]

[82]   Joseph MM, Aswathy G, Manojkumar TK, Sreelekha TT. Galactoxyloglucan-doxorubicin nanoparticles exerts superior cytotoxic effects on cancer cells-A mechanistic and *in silico* approach. Int J Biol Macromol 2016; 92: 20-9.
[http://dx.doi.org/10.1016/j.ijbiomac.2016.06.093] [PMID: 27373427]

[83]   Aravind SR, Joseph MM, Varghese S, Balaram P, Sreelekha TT. Antitumor and immunopotentiating activity of polysaccharide PST001 isolated from the seed Kernel of *Tamarindus indica*: an *in vivo* study in mice. Sci World J 2012.2012361382.
[http://dx.doi.org/10.1100/2012/361382] [PMID: 22593679]

[84]   Sreelekha TT, Vijayakumar T, Ankanthil R, Vijayan KK, Nair MK. Immunomodulatory effects of a polysaccharide from *Tamarindus indica*. Anticancer Drugs 1993; 4(2): 209-12.
[http://dx.doi.org/10.1097/00001813-199304000-00013] [PMID: 8490201]

[85]   Joseph MM, Aravind SR, Varghese S, Mini S, Sreelekha TT. PST-Gold nanoparticle as an effective anticancer agent with immunomodulatory properties. Colloids Surf B Biointerfaces 2013; 104: 32-9.
[http://dx.doi.org/10.1016/j.colsurfb.2012.11.046] [PMID: 23298585]

[86]   Joseph MM, Aravind SR, George SK, Pillai KR, Mini S, Sreelekha TT. Galactoxyloglucan-modified nanocarriers of doxorubicin for improved tumor-targeted drug delivery with minimal toxicity. J Biomed Nanotechnol 2014; 10(11): 3253-68.
[http://dx.doi.org/10.1166/jbn.2014.1957] [PMID: 26000385]

[87]   Aravind SR, Joseph MM, George SK, *et al.* TRAIL-based tumor sensitizing galactoxyloglucan, a novel entity for targeting apoptotic machinery. Int J Biochem Cell Biol 2015; 59: 153-66.
[http://dx.doi.org/10.1016/j.biocel.2014.11.019] [PMID: 25541375]

[88]   Joseph MM, Aravind SR, George SK, Raveendran Pillai K, Mini S, Sreelekha TT. Anticancer activity of galactoxyloglucan polysaccharide-conjugated doxorubicin nanoparticles: Mechanistic insights and interactome analysis. Eur J Pharm Biopharm 2015; 93: 183-95.
[http://dx.doi.org/10.1016/j.ejpb.2015.04.001] [PMID: 25864443]

[89]   Silva FM, Leite MF, Spadaro AC, Uyemura SA, Maistro EL. Assessment of the potential genotoxic risk of medicinal *Tamarindus indica* fruit pulp extract using *in vivo* assays. Genet Mol Res 2009; 8(3): 1085-92.
[http://dx.doi.org/10.4238/vol8-3gmr630] [PMID: 19768670]

[90]   Kobayashi A, Adenan MI, Kajiyama S, Kanzaki H, Kawazu K. A cytotoxic principle of *Tamarindus indica*, di-n-butyl malate and the structure-activity relationship of its analogues. Z Natforsch C J Biosci 1996; 51(3-4): 233-42.
[http://dx.doi.org/10.1515/znc-1996-3-415] [PMID: 8639230]

[91]   Bueno L, Theodorou V, Sekkal S. Xyloglucan: a new agent to protect the intestinal mucosa and to prevent bacterially-mediated alteration of tight junction permeability. United European Gastroenterol J 2014; 2: A591. [Abstract P1675].

[92]   Gnessi L, Bacarea V, Marusteri M, Piqué N. Xyloglucan for the treatment of acute diarrhea: results of a randomized, controlled, open-label, parallel group, multicentre, national clinical trial. BMC

Gastroenterol 2015; 15: 153.
[http://dx.doi.org/10.1186/s12876-015-0386-z] [PMID: 26518158]

[93] Pleşea Condratovici C, Bacarea V, Piqué N. Xyloglucan for the Treatment of Acute Gastroenteritis in Children: Results of a Randomized, Controlled, Clinical Trial. Gastroenterol Res Pract 2016; 20166874207
[http://dx.doi.org/10.1155/2016/6874207] [PMID: 27212943]

[94] Rao PS, Ramanjaneyulu YS, Prisk VR, Schurgers LJ. A Combination of *Tamarindus indica* seeds and *Curcuma longa* Rhizome Extracts Improves Knee Joint Function and Alleviates Pain in Non-Arthritic Adults Following Physical Activity. Int J Med Sci 2019; 16(6): 845-53.
[http://dx.doi.org/10.7150/ijms.32505] [PMID: 31337958]

[95] Iftekhar AS, Rayhan I, Quadir MA, Akhteruzzaman S, Hasnat A. Effect of *Tamarindus indica* fruits on blood pressure and lipid-profile in human model: an *in vivo* approach. Pak J Pharm Sci 2006; 19(2): 125-9.
[PMID: 16751124]

[96] Nyandoi P. Population structure and socio-economic importance of *Tamarindus indica* in Tharaka District. Eastern Kenya 2005.

[97] Khoja AK, Halbe AV. Scope for the use of Tamarind kernel powder as a thickener in textile printing. Man Made Text India 2001; 44: 403-7.

[98] Kumar CS, Bhattacharya S. Tamarind seed: properties, processing and utilization. Crit Rev Food Sci Nutr 2008; 48(1): 1-20.
[http://dx.doi.org/10.1080/10408390600948600] [PMID: 18274963]

[99] Lima DU, Oliveira RC, Buckeridge MS. Seed storage hemicelluloses as wet-end additives in papermaking. Carbohydr Polym 2003; 52: 367-73.
[http://dx.doi.org/10.1016/S0144-8617(03)00008-0]

[100] Soemardji AA. *Tamarindus indica* L. or "Asam Jawa": the sour but sweet and useful Visit Profr Inst Nat Med Univ Toyama Japan 2007; (May): 1-20.

[101] Kumar KPV, Sethuraman MG. Aricanut fibre and tamarind seed coat as raw materials for varnish preparation. Bull Electrochem 2000; 16: 264-6.

[102] Jayaweera DMA. Medicinal plants (Indigenous and exotic) used in Ceylon 1980.

[103] Mahony D. Trees of Somalia: A field guide for development workers. Oxfam GB 1994.

[104] Chungsamarnyart N, Jansawan W. Effect of *Tamarindus indicus* L. against the Boophilus microplus. Kasetsart 2001; 35: 34-9. [Nat Sci].

[105] Naidu A, Chadraprabha MN, Kanamadi RD, Ramachandra TV. Adsorption of methylene blue and amaranth on to tamarind pod shells. J Biochem Technol 2014; 3: 189-92.

[106] Salim AS, Simons AJ, Waruhiu A, Orwa C, Anyango C. Agroforestree database: a tree species reference and selection guide. Nairobi, Kenya: ICRAF 1998.

[107] Sinha RK. Biodiversity conservation through faith and tradition in India: some case studies. Int J Sustain Dev World Ecol 1995; 2: 278-84.
[http://dx.doi.org/10.1080/13504509509469908]

[108] Purseglove JW. Tropical crops. Dicotyledons, Longria Sci Technol 1987; 204-6.

[109] FAO. Low-Income Food-Deficit Countries (LIFDCs) - List for 2018.

[110] Vadivel V, Pugalenthi M. Evaluation of nutritional value and protein quality of an under-utilized tribal food legume. INDIAN J TRADIT KNOW 2010; 9(4): 791-7.

[111] Masette M, Candia A, Ocheng AG. The commercial viability of Tamarind (*Tamarindus indica* L) fruit based products for improved incomes among farmers in Northern and Eastern Uganda. African J Food Sci Technol 2015; 6: 167-76.

[112] Omondi O. Scaling Up the Production and Commercialization of Tamarind Fruit in Kenya: The Missing Value Chain Links Preprints.org 2019.
[http://dx.doi.org/10.20944/preprints201904.0295.v1]

[113] Buyinza M, Muyanja S. Profitability and economic efficacy of Tamarind (*Tamarindus indica* L.) production: A case of Green money in the drylands of Northern Uganda. J Econ Theory 2008; 2: 1-9.

[114] Cunningham A, Ingram W, Howe J, *et al.* Hidden economies, future options: trade in non-timber forest products in eastern indonesia (ACIAR Technical Report 77). 2011.

[115] Buyinza M, Senjonga M, Lusiba B. Economic valuation of a Tamarind (*Tamarindus indica* L.) production system: green money from drylands of eastern Uganda. Small-scale For 2010; 9: 317-29.
[http://dx.doi.org/10.1007/s11842-010-9118-y]

[116] Rivers M, Mark J. *Tamarindus indica*. 2017.https://doi.org/http://dx.doi.org/10.2305/IUCN.UK.2017-3.RLTS.T62020997A62020999.en

[117] Heaton HJ, Whitkus R, Gómez-Pompa A. Extreme ecological and phenotypic differences in the tropical tree chicozapote (*Manilkara zapota* (L.) P. Royen) are not matched by genetic divergence: a random amplified polymorphic DNA (RAPD) analysis. Mol Ecol 1999; 8: 627-32.
[http://dx.doi.org/10.1046/j.1365-294x.1999.00616.x]

[118] Van den Bilcke N, Alaerts K, Ghaffaripour S, Simbo DJ, Samson R. Physico-chemical properties of tamarind (*Tamarindus indica*. L.) fruits from Mali: selection of elite trees for domestication. Genet Resour Crop Evol 2014; 61.
[http://dx.doi.org/10.1007/s10722-014-0080-y]

[119] BGCI. Threat online database. Richmond: Bot. Gard. Conserv. Int 2017.

[120] NAS TL. Resources for the Future. Washingt, DC 1979; pp. 117-21.

CHAPTER 2

Piper nigrum (Black pepper): A Flavor for Health

Bhushan P. Pimple[*], **Amrita M. Kulkarni** and **Ruchita B. Bhor**

P. E. Society's Modern College of Pharmacy, Yamunanagar, Nigdi, Pune, India

Abstract: *Piper nigrum* is an indigenous extensive wine of Piperaceae. It is predominantly cultivated in the humid and subtropical climate of Western Ghats of India, mainly in Konkan and Kerala. The berries of black pepper are developed on axillary catkins. The berries are warty and turn brownish-black on ripening and are strongly aromatic and pungent. The tolerable aroma of the black piper is exploited in culinary preparations across the globe. Traditionally, it is used as a stimulant, antipyretic, analgesic, antiviral, and as a bioavailability enhancer. Consequently, the manifold use of black pepper has augmented its commercial and medicinal importance. Principle ingredients are alkaloids such as piperine, piperlongumine, and piperlonguminine. Recent research proves its beneficial role in the management of hyperlipidemia, obesity, cardiovascular complications, diabetes, *etc*. The proposed chapter will specifically highlight the phytochemical and pharmacological advancements in the research related to *Piper nigrum*.

Keywords: Black pepper, Bioavailability enhancer, *Piper nigrum*.

INTRODUCTION (FIGS. 1 - 3)

Vernacular Names

Hindi: *Pipar, piplamul*

Marathi: *Pimpli*

Tamil: *Kandan, lippilli, pppili, thippili*

Telugu: *Pippallu*

Urdu: *Pippal*

Gujarati*: Pipli*

[*] **Corresponding author Bhushan P. Pimple:** Department of Pharmacognosy, P.E. Society's Modern College of Pharmacy, Yamunanagar, Nigdi, Pune, Maharashtra, India; Tel: +919970830030; E-mail: bhushanppimple@rediffmail.com

Atta-ur-Rahman, M. Iqbal Choudhary & Sammer Yousuf

English: *Black pepper, Jaborandi pepper*

TRADITIONAL CLAIMS [2-6]

• *Piper nigrum* fruits are traditionally used to promote lactation and treat cough in Andaman- Nicobar Islands.

• Brewed *Piper nigrum* was used as a contraceptive in Indonesia.

• Traditional applications of *Piper nigrum* in Assam, India include:

• Bone fractures: *Piper nigrum* seeds, *Cissus quadrangularis* root, *Zingiber perpureum* rhizome, are boiled in water and consumed as juice.

• It is also used in Fever with cold, gastric disturbances, dysmenorrhea, and pneumonia.

• Traditional Moroccan formulation called Msahan includes *Piper nigrum* which is used to treat gynaecological and musculoskeletal disorders.

• Fruits of *Piper nigrum* are used to treat menstrual pain and dog bite in Bangladesh.

DRUG INTERACTIONS

In vitro studies support that piperine increased the sensitivity of Michigan Cancer Foundation-7 (MCF-7) breast cancer cells to paclitaxel (an anticancer drug) [7].

The bioavailability (the amount of drug reaching blood) of fexofenadine (an antihistaminic drug) has been proven to have increased in the presence of piperine. The bioavailability enhancing ability of piperine is attributed to the increased GI emptying in rats [8].

Metabolism or excretion of an anticonvulsant drug, carbamazepine was suppressed during co-administration with piperine resulting in an increase in the bioavailability of carbamazepine [9].

Piperine altered the metabolism of nimesulide (NSAID), by inhibiting the enzyme UDP-glucose dehydrogenase and glucuronidation reaction leading to an increase in the plasma concentration and improving the anti-inflammatory and anti-nociceptive (pain relieving) effects of nimesulide [10].

Decreased levels of antioxidant enzymes, superoxidase dismutase (SOD), catalase (CAT), glutathione reductase (GR), glutathione peroxidase (GPx) and reduced glutathione (GSH) due to benzo(a)pyrene (BaP) toxicity were normalized by curcumin and piperine, thus protecting against oxidative stress Fig. (**4**) [11].

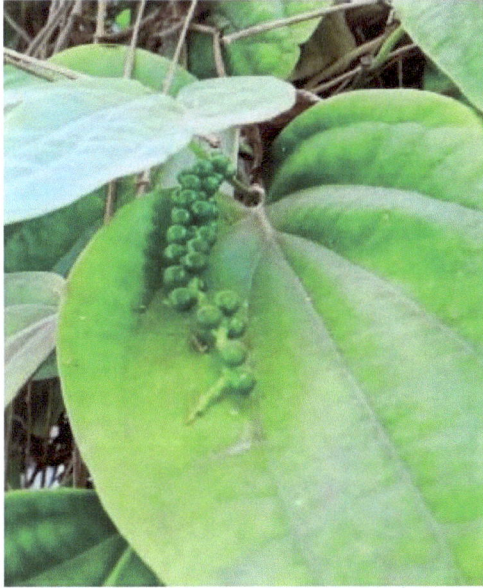

Fig. (1). Catkins of *Piper nigrum*.

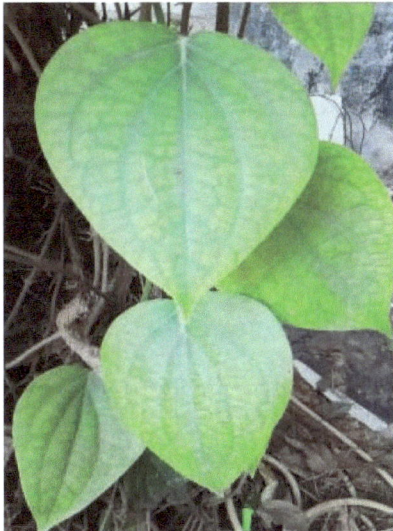

Fig. (2). *Piper nigrum* climber.

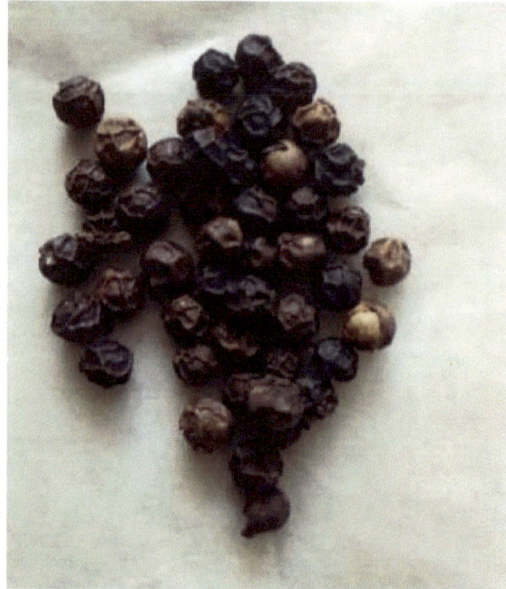

Fig. (3). Dried fruits of *Piper nigrum*.

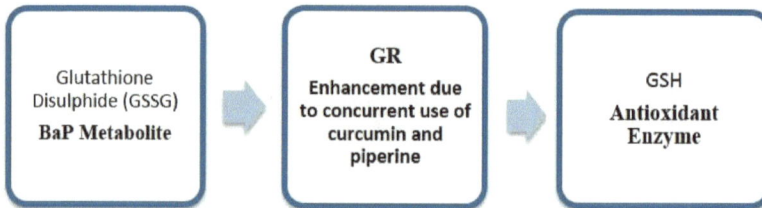

Fig. (4). *Piper nigrum* and oxidative stress.

In vivo studies suggest piperine mediated rise in absorption and delayed elimination of phenytoin (an antiepileptic drug) by altering hepatic first-pass metabolism of phenytoin [12].

Piperine inhibited cytochrome P450 (CYP) metabolic enzymes namely, CYP3A4, CYP2C9 enzymes and decreased the metabolic reactions of Testosterone and Diclofenac [13].

Toxicity Studies of *Piper nigrum*

Convulsions and excitation were the primary symptoms of piperine toxicity in Swiss albino mice and Syrian golden hamsters, irrespective of the route of administration, rapid onset was observed for intravenous (IV) piperine administration, proving IV the most toxic route. Mortality in Fischer rats resulted from haemorrhage (blood loss from the circulatory system) in the stomach, adrenal gland, urinary bladder, small and large intestine at higher doses of piperine [14].

Swiss albino mice treated with pepper extract predominantly developed liver and lung tumours and some developed tumours in the pancreas, thymus, and kidney. The conjoint effect of pepper alkaloids, terpenoids, tannins, safrole in black pepper was attributed to its carcinogenic effect [15].

Piperine caused immunotoxicity in Swiss male mice by decreasing the weight of mesenteric lymph nodes due to its close association with the mesenteric lymph nodes and gut-associated lymphoid tissue (GALT) in the gut, depression in cell population in the thymus and lymph nodes. Higher doses depleted RBCs, leukocytes and haemoglobin contents, antibody-forming cells (AFCs) and maturation of T-cells, thus producing an immunosuppressive effect [16].

The traditional marketed formulations are given in Table **1**.

Table 1. Traditional marketed formulations of *Piper nigrum* [17, 18].

Marketed Formulations	System of Medicine
Marichadi Taila	Ayurvedic
Marichadi Gutika	Ayurvedic
Pippalyadyasava	Ayurvedic
Punarnava guggul	Ayurvedic
Bhaskaralawana churna	Ayurvedic
Madhusnuhi Rasayna	Ayurvedic
Jatiphaladi churna	Ayurvedic
Lohasava	Ayurvedic
Yograj Guggul	Ayurvedic
Goksuradi Guggul	Ayurvedic
Narsimha Guggul	Ayurvedic
Habb-E-Papita Desi	Unani
Habb-E-Tankar	Unani
Jawarish Pudina Wilayti	Unani
Jawarish-E-Bisbasa	Unani
Jawarish-E-Kamooni	Unani
Habb-E-Maghz-E-Badam	Unani

(Table 1) cont.....

Marketed Formulations	System of Medicine
Habb-E-Hindi sual	Unani

GLOBAL AND INDIAN MARKET SIZE

The details of this section are presented in Fig. (**5-8**)

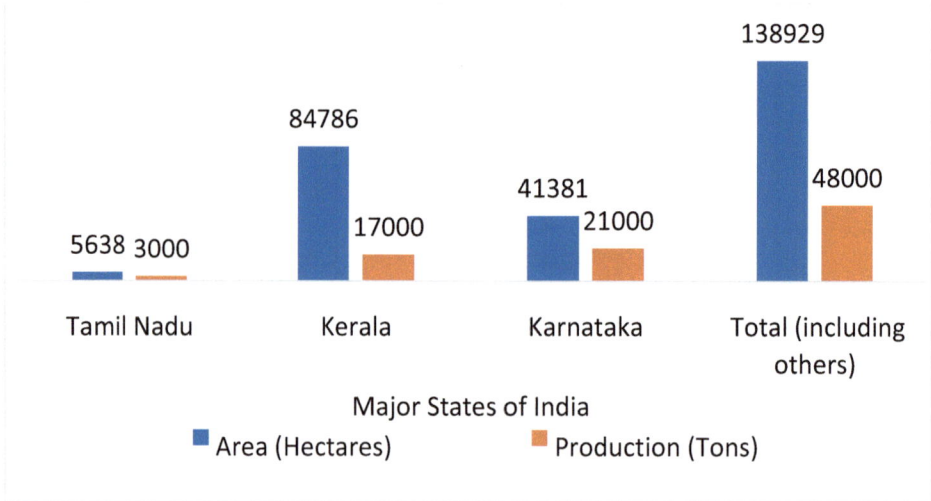

Fig. (5). State-wise and Area and Production Distribution of Pepper in 2018-2019.

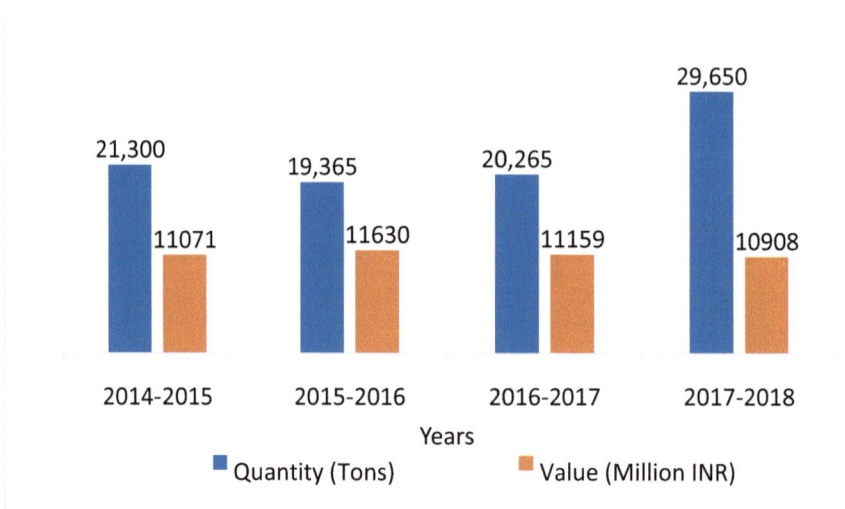

Fig. (6). Pepper Import.

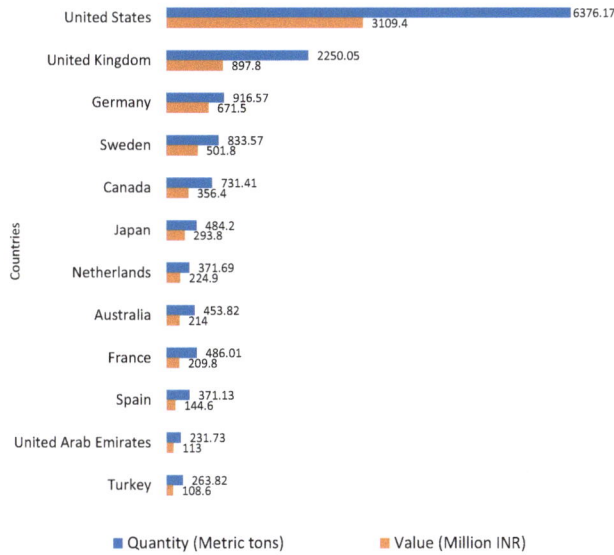

Fig. (7). Country-wise export of pepper from India in 2017-2018 (QTY in M.T; Value in Million INR).

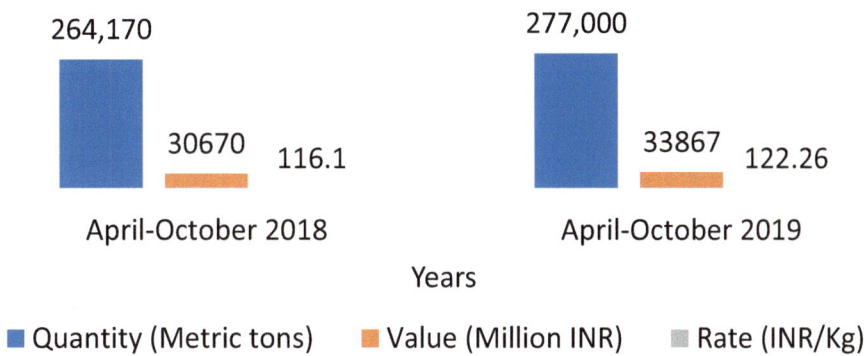

Fig. (8). Estimated export of pepper during April- December 2018 compared with April- December 2019.

PHYTOCHEMISTRY

Reported phytoconstituents of *Piper nigrum* are given in Table **2**.

Table 2. Reported phytoconstituents of *Piper nigrum*.

Class of Phytoconstituents	Phytoconstituents	References
Alkaloids	Piperine, Piperolactum, Paprazine, Sylvamide, Pellitorine, (E)-1-[30,40-(methylenedioxy) cinnamoyl]piperidine, 2,4- tetradecadienoic acid isobutyl amide, Cepharadione.	[20]
Essential oils	α-Pinene Sabinene β-Pinene 3-Carene β-Caryophyllene β-Bisabolene Caryophyllene oxide β-Selinene Monoterpene hydrocarbons Sesquiterpene hydrocarbons Oxygenated sesquiterpenes Oxygenated monoterpenes	[21 - 23]
Phenolic Compounds	Quercetin Isoquercetin Kaempferol-3-o-β-galactoside Kaempferol-3-arabinoside quercetin-3-o-*β*-D rutinoside	[24]
Alkamides	Isopiperolein B Dipiperamide A, B, C Pipercyclobutanamide A, B Retrofractamide C Pipernonaline Piperrolein B Dehydropipernonaline	[25 - 27]

PHARMACOLOGY

Antioxidant

Antioxidant role of methanol extract of *Piper nigrum* alleviated spatial memory deterioration induced by amyloid-beta in the hippocampus of rats [28].

The water and ethanol extracts of *P. nigrum* seeds exhibited potent antioxidant and radical scavenging activities [29].

Essential oils extracted from *Piper nigrum* possessed antioxidant activity by scavenging 1-diphenyl-2-picrylhydrazyl (DPPH) radical [30].

Anti-inflammatory

In vitro anti-inflammatory, nociceptive, and anti-arthritic activity against interleukin 1β (IL1β)-stimulated fibroblast-like synoviocytes (FLSs) derived from patients with rheumatoid arthritis was due to inhibition of the expression of MMP13 (Matrix metalloproteinase 13 gene) in IL1β-stimulated FLSs. Anti-inflammatory and analgesic activity of a higher dose of piperine produced effects similar to prednisolone in rat models of carrageenan-induced acute paw pain and arthritis [31].

Piperine, ethanol, and n-hexane extracts of *P. nigrum* showed anti-inflammatory activity and also exhibited significant analgesic activity in a dose-dependent manner [32].

Piperine exhibited a potent anti-inflammatory effect on 6- OHDA (6-hydroxydopamine) induced Parkinson's disease in Wistar rats by diminishing the inflammatory markers and exhibited neuronal cell protective effect by deactivation of caspase-3 and caspase-9 [33].

Piperine was found to salvage ischemic penumbral region neurons of Wistar rats and limiting the cell death by virtue of its anti-inflammatory activity [34].

Anti-seizure

Piperine exhibited its anti-seizure activity through TRPV1 (Transient receptor potential cation channel subfamily V member 1) receptor in mice, by significantly delaying the onset of myoclonic jerks and generalized clonic seizures [35].

Anti-proliferative and Apoptotic

Piperine inhibited the proliferation of LNCaP, 22RV1, PC-3, and DU-145 prostate cancer cells in a dose-dependent manner. Activation of caspase-3 and cleavage of PARP-1 proteins, induced apoptosis. It disrupted androgen receptor expression and caused a significant diminution in the level of Prostate Specific Antigen in androgen-dependent LNCaP prostate cancer cells. Reduction in the phosphorylation of STAT-3 and Nuclear factor-κB transcription factors reduced prostate cancer proliferation in mice [36].

Piperine suppressed the growth of human rectal adenocarcinoma cells (HRT-18 cells). Concentration and time-dependent cytotoxicity were probably due to a reduction in the number of cells in G2 and M phase of the cell cycle. Piperine induced hydroxyl radical dependent apoptosis. Pre-treatment with antioxidant N-acetylcysteine reduced apoptosis and confirmed the mechanism of cell death [37].

Piperine suppressed the growth of ovarian tumor cells (A2780 cells) barring ovarian epithelial cells by inducing apoptosis in a concentration and time-dependent manner. Apoptosis resulted by activation of caspase 3 and caspase 9 (intracellular proteases) due to proteolytic cleavage of PARP (Poly ADP ribose polymerase). Moreover, the intrinsic apoptotic pathway was confirmed by activation of JNK (c-Jun-N-terminal kinases) and p-38 MAPK (mitogen-activated protein kinase) (apoptotic signalling proteins) [38].

In vitro and *in vivo* studies of piperine on melanoma tumor cells (A375SM and A375P) support cell growth inhibition due to apoptosis. Apoptosis affected due to increased expression of BCL2-associated X (BAX, proapoptotic protein), proteolytic cleavage of PARP and activation of caspase-9 and caspase-3, activation of p-JNK and p-38 MAPK proteins. The decrease in the anti-apoptotic proteins ERK1/2 (phosphoextracellular signal-regulated protein kinase), BCL2 (B-cell lymphoma 2) in a dose-dependent manner was evident [39].

HER2 gene transcription in HER2 overexpressing breast cancer cells was inhibited by piperine thereby inhibited growth and metastasis of the cancer cells. Inhibition of FAS gene and MMP-9 (metallopeptidase 9) expression, PARP cleavage and caspase-3 activation-induced apoptosis. Furthermore, piperine sensitized HER2 overexpressing breast cancer cells to paclitaxel [40].

In vitro cytotoxicity of piperine on human oral squamous carcinoma cells (KB cells) was a result of mitochondrial depolarization, reactive oxygen species and caspase-mediated apoptosis, cell cycle arrest at G0 phase. Nuclear condensation and cell shrinkage caused suppression in tumour growth [41].

Anti-bacterial

Khan *et al.* studied the antibacterial activity of aqueous decoction of *Piper nigrum*, *Laurus nobilis*, *Pimpinella anisum,* and *Coriandum sativum* against different bacterial isolates *Piper nigrum* exhibited strongest antibacterial activity compared to others [42].

Anti-depressant

Piperine administration suppressed depression due to hippocampal neuronal damage induced by corticosterone administration. Antidepressant effects of piperine were due to inhibition of monoaminoxidase enzymes (MAO), regulation of the serotonergic system, and increasing brain-derived neurotrophic factor expression in the hippocampus [43].

Anti-platelet

Rabbit platelet aggregation induced by collagen, arachidonic acid, and platelet-activating factor was inhibited by piperine, pipernonaline, piperoctadecalidine, and piperlongumine. The stronger anti-platelet effect was exhibited by piperlongumine. The pyridone, pyridine, and trimoethoxybenzene groups of piperlongumine may be responsible for the anti-platelet effect against collagen and inhibition of cyclooxygenase (COX) enzyme is responsible for anti-platelet effect against arachidonic acid [44].

Anti-tuberculosis

In vitro immunomodulatory activity of piperine enhanced the efficacy of rifampicin (anti-microbial) against *Mycobacterium tuberculosis* infection in mice. Piperine induced differentiation and proliferation of lymphocytes and Th-1 cytokines and enhanced macrophage activation. Anti-tuberculosis activity was synergistically exhibited by piperine and rifampicin rather than rifampicin alone [45].

Immunomodulatory and Antitumor

Piperine produced cytotoxicity in Ehrlich ascites carcinoma cells, Dalton's lymphoma ascites and L929 cells and suppression of solid tumor growth due to DLA cells. Piperine produced immunomodulation by increasing the total WBC count in Bal b/c mice, increasing the bone marrow cellularity and alpha-esterase positive cells. Immunosuppression due to chemotherapy can be counteracted by piperine administration [46].

Anti-hypertensive

Anti-hypertensive effect was due to the calcium channel blocking effect of piperidine moiety in piperine. Piperine caused a dose-dependent decrease in mean arterial pressure in normotensive rats. *In vitro* antihypertensive effects included partial inhibition of force and rate of ventricular contractions and coronary flow in Langendorrf 's rabbit heart preparation, Ca^{2+} channel blockade in rabbit aortic rings, vasodilation in rat aorta, inhibition of K+ pre contractions in bovine coronary artery preparations [47].

Bioavailability Enhancer

Piperine served as a bioavailability enhancer by altering the membrane dynamics and lipid permeability thereby increasing the absorption and reducing the metabolism by inhibiting drug metabolising enzymes (Cytochrome p450 enzymes, UDP-glucose dehydrogenase (UDP-GDH), aryl hydrocarbon hydroxylase (AAH), and UDP glucuronyl transferase) [48].

CONSENT FOR PUBLICATION

Not applicable.

CONFLICT OF INTEREST

The author declares that there is no conflict of interest in this chapter.

ACKNOWLEDGEMENTS

Declared none.

REFERENCES

[1]   Kumar S, Kamboj J, Suman , Sharma S. Overview for various aspects of the health benefits of *Piper longum* linn. fruit. J Acupunct Meridian Stud 2011; 4(2): 134-40.
[http://dx.doi.org/10.1016/S2005-2901(11)60020-4] [PMID: 21704957]

[2]   Chander MP, Kartick C, Vijayachari P. Ethnomedicinal knowledge among Karens of Andaman & Nicobar Islands, India. J Ethnopharmacol 2015; 162: 127-33.
[http://dx.doi.org/10.1016/j.jep.2014.12.033] [PMID: 25557035]

[3]   Ramdhan B, Chikmawati T, Waluyo EB. Ethnomedical herb from Cikondang indigenous village, district Bandung West Java Indonesia. J Biodivers Environ Sci 2015; 6(2): 277-88.

[4]   Sonowal R, Barua I. Ethnomedical practices among the Tai-Khamyangs of Assam, India. Stud Ethno-Med 2011; 5(1): 41-50.
[http://dx.doi.org/10.1080/09735070.2011.11886390]

[5]   Teixidor-Toneu I, Martin GJ, Ouhammou A, Puri RK, Hawkins JA. An ethnomedicinal survey of a Tashelhit-speaking community in the High Atlas, Morocco. J Ethnopharmacol 2016; 188: 96-110.
[http://dx.doi.org/10.1016/j.jep.2016.05.009] [PMID: 27174082]

[6]   Tumpa SI, Hossain MI, Ishika T. Ethnomedicinal uses of herbs by indigenous medicine practitioners of Jhenaidah district, Bangladesh. J Pharmacogn Phytochem 2014; 3(2): 23-33.

[7]   Motiwala MN, Rangari VD. Combined effect of paclitaxel and piperine on a MCF-7 breast cancer cell line *in vitro*: Evidence of a synergistic interaction. Synergy 2015; 2(1): 1-6.
[http://dx.doi.org/10.1016/j.synres.2015.04.001]

[8]   Jin MJ, Han HK. Effect of piperine, a major component of black pepper, on the intestinal absorption of fexofenadine and its implication on food-drug interaction. J Food Sci 2010; 75(3): H93-6.
[http://dx.doi.org/10.1111/j.1750-3841.2010.01542.x] [PMID: 20492299]

[9]   Pattanaik S, Hota D, Prabhakar S, Kharbanda P, Pandhi P. Pharmacokinetic interaction of single dose of piperine with steady-state carbamazepine in epilepsy patients. Phytother Res 2009; 23(9): 1281-6.
[http://dx.doi.org/10.1002/ptr.2676] [PMID: 19283724]

[10]   Gupta SK, Bansal P, Bhardwaj RK, Velpandian T. Comparative anti-nociceptive, anti-inflammatory and toxicity profile of nimesulide *vs* nimesulide and piperine combination. Pharmacol Res 2000; 41(6): 657-62.
[http://dx.doi.org/10.1006/phrs.1999.0640] [PMID: 10816335]

[11]   Sehgal A, Kumar M, Jain M, Dhawan DK. Piperine as an adjuvant increases the efficacy of curcumin in mitigating benzo(a)pyrene toxicity. Hum Exp Toxicol 2012; 31(5): 473-82.
[http://dx.doi.org/10.1177/0960327111421943] [PMID: 22027502]

[12]   Velpandian T, Jasuja R, Bhardwaj RK, Jaiswal J, Gupta SK. Piperine in food: interference in the pharmacokinetics of phenytoin. Eur J Drug Metab Pharmacokinet 2001; 26(4): 241-7.
[http://dx.doi.org/10.1007/BF03226378] [PMID: 11808866]

[13]   Kimura Y, Ito H, Hatano T. Effects of mace and nutmeg on human cytochrome P450 3A4 and 2C9 activity. Biol Pharm Bull 2010; 33(12): 1977-82.
[http://dx.doi.org/10.1248/bpb.33.1977] [PMID: 21139236]

[14]   Piyachaturawat P, Glinsukon T, Toskulkao C. Acute and subacute toxicity of piperine in mice, rats and hamsters. Toxicol Lett 1983; 16(3-4): 351-9.
[http://dx.doi.org/10.1016/0378-4274(83)90198-4] [PMID: 6857729]

[15]   Concon JM, Newburg DS, Swerczek TW. Black pepper [*Piper nigrum*]: evidence of carcinogenicity

[16]   Dogra RK, Khanna S, Shanker R. Immunotoxicological effects of piperine in mice. Toxicology 2004; 196(3): 229-36.
[http://dx.doi.org/10.1016/j.tox.2003.10.006] [PMID: 15036749]

[17]   Anonymous. The Ayurvedic Pharmacopoeia of India Part-II (formulations) Government of India, Ministry of Health and Family Welfare, Department of Ayurveda, Yoga & Naturopathy, Unani, Siddha and Homoeopathy. 1st ed. 60,70, 107, 112, 121, 123, 157, 175, 200.

[18]   Anonymous The Unani Pharmacopoeia of India, Part – II, Volume - III (Formulations). 1st ed. Government of India Ministry of Ayush, Pharmacopoeia Comission for Indian Medicine & Homoeopathy Ghaziabad. 2016; p. 33,43,51, 57, 61, 65.

[19]   indianspices.com/[Homepage on the internet]. 2019 Spices Board India, Ministry of Commerce & Industry, Govt. of India. Available from: http://indianspices.com/

[20]   Ee GC, Lim CM, Lim CK, Rahmani M, Shaari K, Bong CF. Alkaloids from Piper *sarmentosum* and *Piper nigrum*. Nat Prod Res 2009; 23(15): 1416-23.
[http://dx.doi.org/10.1080/14786410902757998] [PMID: 19809914]

[21]   Kapoor IP, Singh B, Singh G, De Heluani CS, De Lampasona MP, Catalan CA. Chemistry and *in vitro* antioxidant activity of volatile oil and oleoresins of black pepper (*Piper nigrum*). J Agric Food Chem 2009; 57(12): 5358-64.
[http://dx.doi.org/10.1021/jf900642x] [PMID: 19456163]

[22]   Jirovetz L, Buchbauer G, Ngassoum MB, Geissler M. Aroma compound analysis of *Piper nigrum* and Piper guineense essential oils from Cameroon using solid-phase microextraction-gas chromatography, solid-phase microextraction-gas chromatography-mass spectrometry and olfactometry. J Chromatogr A 2002; 976(1-2): 265-75.
[http://dx.doi.org/10.1016/S0021-9673(02)00376-X] [PMID: 12462618]

[23]   Martins AP, Salgueiro L, Vila R, *et al.* Essential oils from four Piper species. Phytochemistry 1998; 49(7): 2019-23.
[http://dx.doi.org/10.1016/S0031-9422(98)00391-4]

[24]   Butt MS, Pasha I, Sultan MT, Randhawa MA, Saeed F, Ahmed W. Black pepper and health claims: a comprehensive treatise. Crit Rev Food Sci Nutr 2013; 53(9): 875-86.
[http://dx.doi.org/10.1080/10408398.2011.571799] [PMID: 23768180]

[25]   Srinivas PV, Rao JM. Isopiperolein B: an alkamide from *Piper nigrum*. Phytochemistry 1999; 52(5): 957-8.
[http://dx.doi.org/10.1016/S0031-9422(99)00287-3]

[26]   Fujiwara Y, Naithou K, Miyazaki T, Hashimoto K, Mori K, Yamamoto Y. Two new alkaloids, pipercyclobutanamides A and B, from *Piper nigrum*. Tetrahedron Lett 2001; 42(13): 2497-9.

[http://dx.doi.org/10.1016/S0040-4039(01)00209-X]

[27]   Lee SW, Rho MC, Park HR, *et al.* Inhibition of diacylglycerol acyltransferase by alkamides isolated from the fruits of *Piper longum* and *Piper nigrum*. J Agric Food Chem 2006; 54(26): 9759-63.
[http://dx.doi.org/10.1021/jf061402e] [PMID: 17177498]

[28]   Hritcu L, Noumedem JA, Cioanca O, Hancianu M, Kuete V, Mihasan M. Methanolic extract of *Piper nigrum* fruits improves memory impairment by decreasing brain oxidative stress in amyloid beta(1-42) rat model of Alzheimer's disease. Cell Mol Neurobiol 2014; 34(3): 437-49.
[http://dx.doi.org/10.1007/s10571-014-0028-y] [PMID: 24442916]

[29]   Gülçin I. The antioxidant and radical scavenging activities of black pepper (*Piper nigrum*) seeds. Int J Food Sci Nutr 2005; 56(7): 491-9.
[http://dx.doi.org/10.1080/09637480500450248] [PMID: 16503560]

[30]   Bagheri H, Abdul Manap MY, Solati Z. Antioxidant activity of *Piper nigrum* L. essential oil extracted by supercritical CO_2 extraction and hydro-distillation. Talanta 2014; 121: 220-8.
[http://dx.doi.org/10.1016/j.talanta.2014.01.007] [PMID: 24607131]

[31]   Bang JS, Oh DH, Choi HM, *et al.* Anti-inflammatory and antiarthritic effects of piperine in human interleukin 1β-stimulated fibroblast-like synoviocytes and in rat arthritis models. Arthritis Res Ther 2009; 11(2): R49.
[http://dx.doi.org/10.1186/ar2662] [PMID: 19327174]

[32]   Tasleem F, Azhar I, Ali SN, Perveen S, Mahmood ZA. Analgesic and anti-inflammatory activities of *Piper nigrum* L. Asian Pac J Trop Med 2014; 7S1: S461-8.
[http://dx.doi.org/10.1016/S1995-7645(14)60275-3] [PMID: 25312168]

[33]   Shrivastava P, Vaibhav K, Tabassum R, *et al.* Anti-apoptotic and anti-inflammatory effect of Piperine on 6-OHDA induced Parkinson's rat model. J Nutr Biochem 2013; 24(4): 680-7.
[http://dx.doi.org/10.1016/j.jnutbio.2012.03.018] [PMID: 22819561]

[34]   Vaibhav K, Shrivastava P, Javed H, *et al.* Piperine suppresses cerebral ischemia-reperfusion-induced inflammation through the repression of COX-2, NOS-2, and NF-κB in middle cerebral artery occlusion rat model. Mol Cell Biochem 2012; 367(1-2): 73-84.
[http://dx.doi.org/10.1007/s11010-012-1321-z] [PMID: 22669728]

[35]   Chen CY, Li W, Qu KP, Chen CR. Piperine exerts anti-seizure effects *via* the TRPV1 receptor in mice. Eur J Pharmacol 2013; 714(1-3): 288-94.
[http://dx.doi.org/10.1016/j.ejphar.2013.07.041] [PMID: 23911889]

[36]   Samykutty A, Shetty AV, Dakshinamoorthy G, *et al.* Piperine, a bioactive component of pepper spice exerts therapeutic effects on androgen dependent and androgen independent prostate cancer cells. PLoS One 2013; 8(6)e65889
[http://dx.doi.org/10.1371/journal.pone.0065889] [PMID: 23824300]

[37]   Yaffe PB, Doucette CD, Walsh M, Hoskin DW. Piperine impairs cell cycle progression and causes reactive oxygen species-dependent apoptosis in rectal cancer cells. Exp Mol Pathol 2013; 94(1): 109-14.
[http://dx.doi.org/10.1016/j.yexmp.2012.10.008] [PMID: 23063564]

[38]   Si L, Yang R, Lin R, Yang S. Piperine functions as a tumor suppressor for human ovarian tumor growth *via* activation of JNK/p38 MAPK-mediated intrinsic apoptotic pathway. Biosci Rep 2018; 38(3)BSR20180503
[http://dx.doi.org/10.1042/BSR20180503] [PMID: 29717031]

[39]   Yoo ES, Choo GS, Kim SH, *et al.* Antitumor and apoptosis-inducing effects of piperine on human melanoma cells. Anticancer Res 2019; 39(4): 1883-92.
[http://dx.doi.org/10.21873/anticanres.13296] [PMID: 30952729]

[40]   Do MT, Kim HG, Choi JH, *et al.* Antitumor efficacy of piperine in the treatment of human HER2-overexpressing breast cancer cells. Food Chem 2013; 141(3): 2591-9.

[http://dx.doi.org/10.1016/j.foodchem.2013.04.125] [PMID: 23870999]

[41]   Siddiqui S, Ahamad MS, Jafri A, Afzal M, Arshad M. Piperine triggers apoptosis of human oral squamous carcinoma through cell cycle arrest and mitochondrial oxidative stress. Nutr Cancer 2017; 69(5): 791-9.
[http://dx.doi.org/10.1080/01635581.2017.1310260] [PMID: 28426244]

[42]   Rahman S, Parvez AK, Islam R, Khan MH. Antibacterial activity of natural spices on multiple drug resistant *Escherichia coli* isolated from drinking water, Bangladesh. Ann Clin Microbiol Antimicrob 2011; 10(1): 10.
[http://dx.doi.org/10.1186/1476-0711-10-10] [PMID: 21406097]

[43]   Mao QQ, Huang Z, Zhong XM, Xian YF, Ip SP. Piperine reverses the effects of corticosterone on behavior and hippocampal BDNF expression in mice. Neurochem Int 2014; 74: 36-41.
[http://dx.doi.org/10.1016/j.neuint.2014.04.017] [PMID: 24816193]

[44]   Park BS, Son DJ, Park YH, Kim TW, Lee SE. Antiplatelet effects of acidamides isolated from the fruits of Piper longum L. Phytomedicine 2007; 14(12): 853-5.
[http://dx.doi.org/10.1016/j.phymed.2007.06.011] [PMID: 17689230]

[45]   Sharma S, Kalia NP, Suden P, *et al.* Protective efficacy of piperine against *Mycobacterium tuberculosis*. Tuberculosis (Edinb) 2014; 94(4): 389-96.
[http://dx.doi.org/10.1016/j.tube.2014.04.007] [PMID: 24880706]

[46]   Sunila ES, Kuttan G. Immunomodulatory and antitumor activity of Piper longum Linn. and piperine. J Ethnopharmacol 2004; 90(2-3): 339-46.
[http://dx.doi.org/10.1016/j.jep.2003.10.016] [PMID: 15013199]

[47]   Taqvi SI, Shah AJ, Gilani AH. Blood pressure lowering and vasomodulator effects of piperine. J Cardiovasc Pharmacol 2008; 52(5): 452-8.
[http://dx.doi.org/10.1097/FJC.0b013e31818d07c0] [PMID: 19033825]

[48]   Acharya SG, Momin AH, Gajjar AV. Review of piperine as a bio-enhancer. Am J Pharm Tech Res 2012; 2: 32-44.

CHAPTER 3

Coriander Seeds: Ethno-medicinal, Phytochemical and Pharmacological Profile

Samra Bashir[*] and **Asif Safdar**

Department of Pharmacy, Capital University of Science and Technology, Islamabad, Pakistan

Abstract: Coriander (*Coriandrum sativum* L.; family Apiaceae/Umbelliferae), locally known as dhanya, is a popular culinary herb, well recognized for its therapeutic properties in Indo-Pak subcontinent. The plant is native to North Africa, Southern Europe, and southwestern Asia and is also one of the widely cultivated herbs. The aerial plant parts including seeds of coriander are being excessively used in traditional cuisines due to its pleasant color and flavor. Coriander seeds are commonly used spices and ingredients of curry and traditional recipes in the Mediterranean and South Asian regions.

The leaves (hara dhanya) are also used to garnish meals before serving. Besides, essential oils of coriander leaves and seeds are also used in several foods including fish and meat products, beverages, pickles, and sweets due to its pleasant aroma and health benefits owing to high free radical scavenging activity. Apart from culinary applications, coriander seeds and leaves are also well recognized for their therapeutic potential in traditional medicine since ages. Coriander is known to have significant hypoglycemic, hypo-cholesterolemic, anti-inflammatory, hepato-protective, and antioncogenic potential. It is also effective in mitigating gastrointestinal complications.

Keywords: Apiaceae/Umbelliferae, Antimicrobial, *Coriandrum sativum*, Culinary herb, Ethno-medicinal uses, Essential oil, Phytochemistry, Petroselinic acid, Pharmacology.

INTRODUCTION

Herbs and spices are known for their curative and disease preventive potential since time immemorial. The healthful effects of these natural remedies have been attributed to the presence of secondary metabolites commonly ascribed as phytochemicals. These plant constituents belong to diverse chemical classes of compounds, including alkaloids, polyphenols, sterols, tannins, and terpenoids and are attributed with a range of medicinal effects, also known as bioactivity. A sign-

---

[*] **Corresponding author Samra Bashir:** Department of Pharmacy, Capital University of Science and Technology, Islamabad, Pakistan; Tel: 0092-333-2549700 E-mail: samrabashir@gmail.com

Atta-ur-Rahman, M. Iqbal Choudhary & Sammer Yousuf

ificant proportion of the world population relies on these herb-based remedies for their health care needs.

Coriander (locally known as dhaniya) is one of the oldest known herbs and has been utilized for over 3000 years for both medicinal and therapeutic purposes. Although native to the mediterranean region, coriander is globally cultivated in Asia, North Africa, and Central Europe. Coriander is a well-known and widely cultivated herb due to its culinary value and therapeutic effects [1]. The aerial part of the plant including leaves, stem, and coriander fruit possesses pleasant flavor and aroma, making it a popular spice and ingredient of traditional cuisine. Besides, leaves and seeds of coriander have been used in traditional medicines including Unani and Ayurveda for diverse therapeutic applications for ages. The medicinal effects reported in coriander seeds and herb include anti-inflammatory, anti-hypercholesterolemic, hypoglycemic, hepatoprotective, and antioncogenic activities [2]. Additionally, coriander is also effective in relieving gastrointestinal complaints including diarrhea, anorexia, flatulence, dyspepsia, and vomiting. Variable quantities of fats, proteins, carbohydrates, minerals, fibers, and vitamins are present among constituents of coriander.

ARCHEO-BOTANICAL DESCRIPTION

As evident from the written history, coriander is one of the oldest spices; however, the origin of the cultivated as well as wild species is still not clear. The oldest archaeological remains of the crop date to around 6000 BC in Israel and Palestine [3]. The plant has since spread throughout the world, and different strains of the plant have developed. Coriander as a medicinal plant is listed in an Egyptian papyrus dated from 1550 BC [4]. It is interesting to note that the ancient Egyptian literature mentions varieties of coriander coming from Asia [5]. Coriander fruits were found in the tomb of Tutankhamun and other ancient Egyptian graves at that time [5]. The Greek literature by Aristophanes, Theophrastus, Hippocrates, and Dioscorides also mentioned this crop. Egyptian coriander was especially praised by them for its quality. The word "Coriandrum" also has its origin from ancient Greek which means bed bug-like smell. In China, coriander is mentioned as a vegetable in a book on agriculture from the 5th century [6]. The Persian name for coriander was used in China, which lends support to the hypothesis that the plant was introduced to China from this area. The old Russian name 'ki nec' is very similar to the Persian 'geshnes' and Turkish 'kisnis', and the crop probably came to Russia from the Caucasus or even from areas to the east of the Caspian Sea. Coriander reached South-East Asia from two routes: ovoid fruit-bearing varieties were introduced from India, while those with small, globular fruits arrived later (after 400 AD) from China [5].

The height of the plant can vary between 20 and 120 cm, depending upon the agro-climatic conditions. The whole plant of coriander, including fruits/seeds, leaves, stem, and roots possess aromatic odor and flavor. Leaves are pinnately or ternately decompound, lower ones long petioled and upper ones short petioled. Only young leaves, not yet divided into narrow linear segments, are used to flavor sauces and curries. The plant has thin, spindle-shaped roots. The thin erect stalk is sympodial, monochasial and branched with several side branches at the basal node. In the flowering season, each branch gives off an inflorescence. The flowers are small, in compound terminal umbels, and white or pinkish purple in colour. The ripe fruits/seeds are yellowish-brown globular or ovate, consisting of two pericarps, with a diameter up to 4-5 mm.

The seed essential oil that gives the plant its characteristic "bug" smell lies inside the convex longitudinal vittae. The odor characteristics of different parts of the plant change dramatically as a result of maturity. Ripe fruits smell differently from the unripe seeds and green leaves [7, 8]. The ripe seeds of the plant are shown in Fig. (**1**).

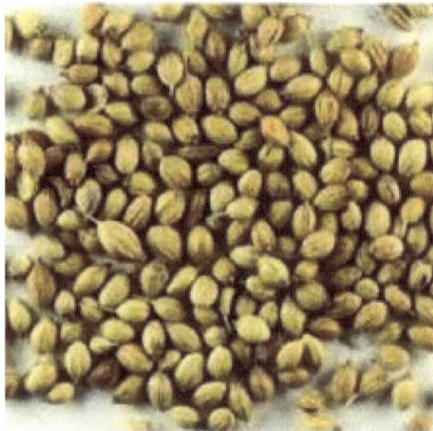

Fig. (1). Seeds of coriander (*Coriandrum sativum* L.).

PLANT TAXONOMY, DISTRIBUTION, AND CULTIVATION

Coriander (*Coriandrum sativum* L.) belongs to the carrot family Apiceae/Umbelliferae and, along with the wild species, *C. tordylium*, is a member of the genus *Coriandrum* [9].

Coriander, a native of Italy, is presently cultivated in Central and Eastern Europe, Mediterranean regions (Morocco, Malta, Egypt), and Asia (China, Russia, Pakistan, India, and Bangladesh), as a spice, or for essential oil production.

Coriander is an annual herbaceous plant but grows best in the cold season between October and February. Flowering occurs between June and July. It is generally cultivated on black soil and rich silt loam requiring no or minimum irrigation. Germination starts 10 to 25 days after sowing the fruit halves. The plant flowers after 40-60 days of sowing and the fruit get fully ripe and are ready to harvest in 3-4 months time [10, 11]. Different growth stages of coriander are shown in Fig. (2).

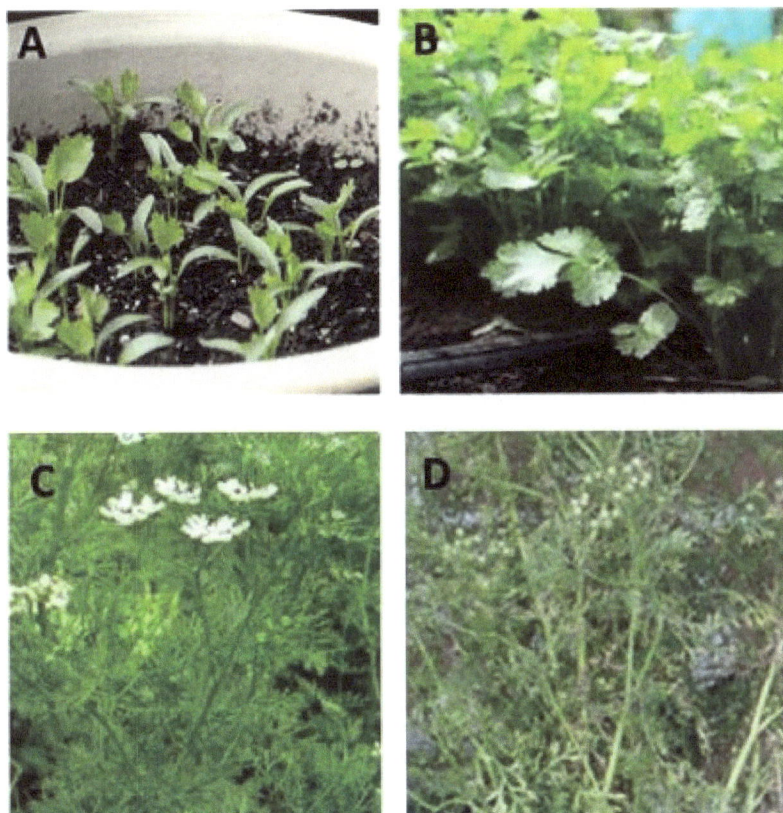

Fig. (2). Different growth stages of coriander (*Coriandrum sativum* L): **A.** coriander seedlings, **B.** young plant, **C.** flowering stage, **D.** fruit-bearing stage.

CORIANDER: ETHNO-MEDICINAL USES

All parts of the coriander plant including the leaves, seeds, root, stem, and essential oil have been used for both dietary and therapeutic purposes [1]. The leaves and seeds of coriander, exhibiting pleasant aroma and flavor, are a popular spice and are used to garnish and flavor traditional cuisine in the Mediterranean region and Subcontinent [12]. The root part of the plant is generally used in a range of Asian foods while the chopped stem of coriander is mostly utilized in stews and soups preparation [13]. Alongside its culinary value, coriander is a popular traditional remedy for the prevention and treatment of various diseases in indigenous medicinal systems of diverse societies. The leaves have been used as an antispasmodic, dyspeptic, appetizer and to treat abdominal discomforts. Herbal preparations constituting of coriander leaves are ingested or applied externally to relieve inflammation in arthritis and rheumatism, indigestion as a carminative agent, cough, bronchitis, vomiting, dysentery, diarrhea, gout, rheumatism, intermittent fevers and giddiness among others [14]. Antiedemic, antiseptic, emmenagogue, and nerve soothing are among other uses attributed to coriander leaves [2]. In Pakistan, the whole coriander plant is a popular folk remedy for the treatment of diarrhea, dysentery, flatulence, jaundice, vomiting, and stomach problems [15]. It is also used as an analgesic, diuretic, refrigerant, and tonic all over the country.

The Indian traditional system widely employs coriander to cure digestive, respiratory, and urinary systems ailment as well as utilizes it as carminative, diuretic, diaphoretic, and stimulant. Brewed coriander seeds have been utilized in Turkey as a carminative, digestive aid, and appetite enhancer [16]. The seeds are combined with caraway and cardamom seeds or with caraway, fennel, and anise seeds in eastern medicine practiced in Pakistan to treat digestive complaints.

In traditional Chinese medicine (TCM), coriander seeds are administered to treat indigestion, anorexia, stomach ache, influenza with no sweating, bad breath, and unpleasant odors from genital areas [17], whereas, in Germany, coriander seeds are usually taken as medicinal teas or components of carminatives and laxatives. The main use is to treat anorexia, dyspepsia, and gastrointestinal discomforts. The fruit is listed in the European Pharmacopoeias and is used as a digestive aid, against worms and to treat rheumatism. In Iran, coriander has a long history of medicinal use for preventing convulsions, anxiety, insomnia, and loss of appetite. The essential oil from the coriander plant has also been used traditionally in the Asian region to stimulate gastric secretion and treat gastric ulcers, and mouth infections [17, 18].

Coriander is also a folk medicine for the treatment of hyperglycemia in some countries like Jordan, Morocco, Saudi Arabia, and Iran [19 - 21]. Ayurvedic literature has endorsed the efficacy of regular consumption of coriander seeds in lowering the serum lipid levels, whereas, the utilization of coriander as a treatment of urinary infections and diuretic has been recorded by Moroccan and Palestinian pharmacopeias [22, 23]. A significant proportion of the population still uses an infusion of coriander seeds as an anti-diabetic agent in Saudi Arabia [19], and the seed extract has been used to decrease fertility [24]. Additionally, formulations containing coriander as principal constituent such as "Maharasnadhi Quather" have long been recommended by Ayurvedic practitioners to treat arthritis and inflammations.

In traditional Iranian medicine, coriander is a time tested treatment for anxiety, convulsions, and insomnia. It has also been employed as an antimicrobial, antiseptic, and wound-healing agent in the mouth. Coriander is a conventional measure to cure cough and bronchitis [16].

PHYTOCHEMISTRY OF CORIANDER SEED

Coriander seeds are the most widely used components of the plant. The most important constituents of the seeds include the essential oil and the fixed/fatty oil. The fixed oil composition of the seed is around 25%, whereas the essential oil constitutes less than 1% of the coriander seed.

Fatty Oil

The light yellow colored fatty oil of coriander is with a characteristic odor. The components of coriander fatty oil have been well studied and are classified into lipids and sterols. Neutral lipids are a major faction of the total lipids (93 to 95.65%) and are majorly composed of triglycerides (95.50%), diacylglycerols (1.88%), and free fatty acids (2.05%). Glycolipids and phospholipids constitute 4.14 and 1.57% of the fatty oil, respectively. The predominant fatty acids highlighted in coriander seed is petroselinic acid present in the concentration of about 65.70–80.9% trailed by linoleic acid, 13.0–16.7%. Other FAs include oleic acid, palmitic acid, and stearic acid. Furthermore, palmitoleic (0.4–1.1%), α-linolenic (0.15–0.50%), and arachidic (0.10–0.25%) were also identified in lesser quantities, as shown in Table **1** [25].

Table 1. Maximum fatty acid composition of coriander (*Coriandrum sativum* L.) seeds of different origins.

Chemical Constituent	Percentage	Region	Extraction Method (if any)	Reference
C14:0 (myristic acid)	0.08	Korba (North-Eastern Tunisia)	hydro-distillation	[29]
C16:0 (palmitic acid)	3.96	Germany	hydro-distillation	[29]
C18:0 (stearic acid)	2.91 & 0.7	Germany & Charfine (North-Eastern Tunisia)	hydro-distillation	[25]
C20:0 (arachidic acid)	0.25	Germany	hydro-distillation	[29]
C16:1n-7 (palmitoleic acid)	0.41	Germany	hydro-distillation	[29]

(Table 1) cont.....

Chemical Constituent	Percentage	Region	Extraction Method (if any)	Reference
C18: 1n-9 (oleic acid)	7.85	Germany	hydro-distillation	[29]
C18:1n-12 (petroselinic acid)	80.9	Charfine (north-eastern Tunisia)	hydro-distillation	[25]
C18: 2n-6 (linoleic acid)	16.7	Germany	hydro-distillation	[29]
C18: 3n-3 (α-linolenic acid)	0.20	Germany	hydro-distillation	[29]
C18: 3n-6 (γ-linolenic acid)	1.22	Germany	hydro-distillation	[29]
C20: 1n-9 (gadoleic acid)	0.30	Germany	hydro-distillation	[29]
C22:6n-3 (docosahexenoic acid)	0.34	Germany	hydro-distillation	[29]

Major phospholipids in coriander fixed oil include phosphatidylcholine (35.98%), followed by 33.83% phosphatidylethanolamine and 15.40% phosphatidylinositol. Whereas, phosphatidic acid (8.11%) and phosphatidylglycerol (6.68%) have been detected in a lesser amount. The most abundant galactolipid detected in coriander oil is digalactosyldiacylglycerol (62.32%), followed by onogalactosyldiacyl-glycerol (37.68%) [26].

The seed oil of coriander has been recognized as an essential source of sterols. Previous studies have reported the total sterol content in a range of 36.93–51.86 mg/ gram of oil. The most common sterols are β-sitosterol and stigmasterol, respectively, constituting 24.8–36.8% and 36.93–51.86 mg/g of coriander oil. Other characteristic sterols are Δ5- and Δ7-stigmasterol, campesterol, and 24-stigmastadienol, whereas, Δ5-avenasterol and Δ7-avenasterol exist in lower quantities.

Seed oil from the Tunisian variety of coriander seeds is identified to contain a small amount of cholesterol *i.e.*, 1.02–2.18% [27]. Nonetheless, two other sterols named lanosterol and ergosterol have been detected in the German variety [28].

Coriander seeds have also been proved as a rich source of tocols which are about 327.47 μg/g of the oil. The chief tocopherol is γ-tocopherol (26.40 mg/g), followed by δ -tocopherol (13.5–36.5 mg/g) and α-tocopherol (6–11.7 mg/g). The seed oil also contains tocotrienols where γ -tocotrienol is the main compound (238.40 mg/g), followed by α -tocotrienol (24.9 mg/g) and δ -tocotrienol (12.57 mg/g) [29].

Composition of Essential Oil

Essential oils are a well-recognized source of bioactive constituents with potential health benefits [30]. A number of researchers across the world have investigated the essential oil content of coriander seed and its composition (Table 2). Steam and hydrodistillation are commonly used methods for the extraction of volatile oil from coriander seeds. The seed essential oil yield is around 1%, with some variation based on climatic conditions and geographical location. Among constituents isolated from coriander essential oil, alcoholic monoterpenes predominately (S)-(þ)-linalool has been identified as the major bioactive constituent (37.67 to 87.54% of the total essential oil), followed by monoterpene hydrocarbons (8.00%). Additional constituents identified in the essential oil from serval coriander varieties include cis-dihydrocarvone, p-mentha-1,4-dien-7-ol, neryl acetate, and α-pinene, neryl acetate, γ-terpinene, and geranyl acetate The content of linalool in the essential oil of the coriander seeds of Pakistani origin was about 69.60%; other bioactive components were geranyl acetate α-pinene, γ-terpinene, anethole, and p-cymene found in considerable quantities as 4.99%, 1.63%, 4.17%, 1.15%, and 1.12%, respectively [31]. Coriander variety from Atlantic Canada exhibited the presence of some additional constituents including camphor, phellandrene, linalyl acetate, limonene, and paracymene [32], whereas geraniol and (Z)-isoapiole have been reported in Turkish varieties in addition to the contents reported in other coriander varieties [33].

Table 2. Essential oil composition (%) of coriander (*Coriandrum sativum* L.) Seeds from different origins.

Chemical Constituent	Percentage	Region	Extraction Method (if any)	Reference
α-Pinene	4.09	India	hydro-distillation	[34]
β-Pinene	1.82	Bangladesh	hydro-distillation	[35]
γ-Terpinene	14.42	Bangladesh	hydro-distillation	[35]
α-Cedrene	3.87	Bangladesh	hydro-distillation	[35]
α-Farnasene	1.22	Bangladesh	hydro-distillation	[35]
p-Cymene	2.16	Brazil	hydro-distillation	[36]
Limonene	1.28	Brazil	hydro-distillation	[36]
Linalool	87.54	Tunisia	hydro-distillation	[37]
Citronellal	1.96	Bangladesh	hydro-distillation	[35]
Camphor	3.4-6.2	Atlantic Canada	hydro-distillation	[32]
Geraniol	1.87	Bangladesh	hydro-distillation	[35]
Anethole	1.15	Pakistan	hydro-distillation	[31]

(Table 2) cont.....

Chemical Constituent	Percentage	Region	Extraction Method (if any)	Reference
Cis-dihydrocarvone	2.36	Tunisia	hydro-distillation	[37]
p-Mentha-1,4-dien-7-ol	6.51	Algeria	hydro-distillation	[38]
Geranyl acetate	17.57	Bangladesh	hydro-distillation	[35]
Neryl acetate	3.22	Algeria	hydro-distillation	[38]
Linalyl-acetate	2.4-3.3	Atlantic Canada	hydro-distillation	[38]
Phellandrene	1.7-4.1	Atlantic Canada	hydro-distillation	[38]
(E)-2-Decenal	0.1-0.6	Iran	hydro-distillation	[39]
Decanal	0.43	Algeria	hydro-distillation	[38]

Polyphenols

Around 21 components have been identified from seeds extracts of various coriander varieties including 11 phenolic acids: chlorogenic, gallic, vanillic, caffeic, p-coumaric, rosmarinic, ferulic, o-coumaric, salicylic, trans-hydroxycinnamic, and trans-cinnamic acids and almost 10 flavonoids identified as quercetin-3-rhamnoside, luteolin, rutin trihydrate, resorcinol, quercetin dihydrate, kaempferol, apigenin, naringin, coumarin, and flavone.

Moreover, it was elucidated that among the derivatives, caffeoyl N-tryptophan hexoside was the most abundant phenolic derivative present at a concentration level of about 45.33 mg/kg, while caffeoyl N-tryptophan was among the least abundant derivatives as depicted from the concentration, *i.e.*, 0.71 mg/kg, in the methanolic extracts of coriander seeds [40].

Additionally, the whole composition of polyphenol of seeds includes feruloyl N-tryptophan hexoside, p-coumaric acid, ferulic acid, feruloyl N-tryptophan, caffeic acid, di-*O*-caffeoylquinic acid, 3-*O*-caffeoylquinic acid, and ferulic acid derivatives [40]. In addition, coriander possesses an appreciable amount of β-carotene and carotenoid, correspondingly [41].

Glycosides

A few studies have reported the presence of four novel monoterpenoid glycosides, two monoterpenoid glucoside sulfates, and two novel aromatic compound glycosides have been reported as water-soluble constituents in coriander seed. Other two glycosides 2-C- methyl-D- erythritol were isolated from coriander seeds [42].

SCIENTIFIC STUDIES ON CORIANDER

Anti-microbial Activity

Several reports have indicated that essential oil and extracts of coriander seeds have potential natural anti-microbial activities [43 - 46]. The essential oil extracted from coriander seeds has shown inhibitory activity against many bacteria and fungi species. The essential oil caused marked inhibition of both Gram-positive (*e.g. Staphylococcus aureus* and *Bacillus spp*) and Gram-negative bacteria (*e.g. Escherichia coli, Pseudomonas aeruginosa, Salmonella typhi, Klebsiella pneumonia,* and *Proteus mirabilis*). The essential oil from seed also exhibited antifungal activity against *Candida albicans.*

The antimicrobial activity exhibited by various chemical fractions of the essential oil was found comparable to the standard antibiotics [45 - 47]. In another study by Singh *et al.* [34] using the inverted plate method, the essential oil was found very active against fungal species including *C. palliscens, F. oxysporum, F. moniliforme,* and *A. terreus*, with more than 70% zone of inhibition. The poisoned food technique showed 100% inhibition of *A. terreus, A. niger, F. graminearum,* and *F. oxysporum* by the essential oil. Traditionally, coriander has been used as an antimicrobial, antiseptic, and wound-healing agent in mouth, although coriander aqueous decoction has shown no antibacterial potential against almost 176 isolates of bacteria originated from 12 distinct genera of bacterial colonies obtained from the oral cavity of 200 individuals by means of disc diffusion technique [48].

Antioxidant Activity

The enormous antioxidant potential of coriander seeds has widely been revealed through several scientific studies. In an early study, the administration of coriander seeds in rats fed with a high-fat diet decreased peroxides, free fatty acids, and glutathione levels as well as increased activity of antioxidant enzymes [49]. In another study, the antioxidant activity of extracts of different polarity from coriander leaves and seeds as well as coriander oil was evaluated by three different methods including diphenyl picrylhydrazyl (DPPH) radical scavenging activity, inhibition of 15-lipoxygenase (15-LO), and inhibition of Fe^{2+}-induced peroxidation of the porcine brain [50]. Ethyl acetate extract, bearing a medium polarity, showed a strong antioxidant activity when assessed by DPPH radical scavenging. Ethanolic extracts inhibited 15-LO in a concentration-dependent manner, with the leaves being more active than the seeds, while lipophilic extracts and coriander oil were found inactive. There was no activity observed in the phospholipid (PL) peroxidation method. Coriander seed oil caused 35% and 32.4% scavenging of DPPH and galvinoxyl radicals, respectively. This free radical scavenging activity of coriander was found higher than black cumin and Niger crude seed oil. The radical scavenging activity of coriander oil has been partly attributed to the high composition of unsaponifiables (21.8 g/kg), and PL present in coriander seed oil [51]. Recently, considerable interest has been shown towards improving the nutritional and functional properties of cooking oils through blending with some non-conventional oils. In 2012, Ramadan and Wahdan [52] explored the effect of blending coriander seed oil with corn oil and assessed the functionality, stability, and radical scavenging activity of the oil blends produced. Corn oil blended with coriander oil (at proportion 10–20%) showed enhanced oxidative stability and DPPH free radical scavenging capacity as compared to corn oil. This improvement in oxidation parameters and antioxidant attributes of oil blend was supposed to be attributed to positive changes in the FA and tocopherols profiles as well as the presence of bioactive compounds such as ST and tocols in coriander seed oil. Similarly, oxidative stability of high linoleic sunflower oil, when blended with coriander seed oil, was also improved as a result of a decrease in linoleic acid and an increase in tocols levels of the blend. The improvement effect was found to be dose-dependent [53]. The effect of polyphenolic extract of coriander seeds was assessed on hydrogen peroxide (H_2O_2)-induced oxidative stress in human lymphocytes [54]. Treatment with H_2O_2 caused oxidative stress by decreasing activities of antioxidant enzymes (*i.e.* superoxide dismutase 'SOD', catalase 'CAT', glutathione peroxidase 'GOP', glutathione reductase 'GR', and glutathione-S-transferase). A general decrease in glutathione content and an increase in thiobarbituric acid-reactive substances (TBARS) was observed. Treatment with polyphenolic fractions of coriander seeds (50 mg/mL) effectively protected human lymphocytes from H_2O_2-induced oxidative stress and restored oxidative stress to that of normal cells. There was an increase in the activities of the antioxidant enzymes and glutathione content, and TBARS content was decreased. The protective effect was comparable to that of a pure compound, quercetin, a known antioxidant [54]. There is supporting evidence that coriander possesses hepatoprotective activity against carbon tetrachloride (CCl_4) intoxication *in vivo* [55]. There was a significant decrease in liver weight and other biomarker elements such as aspartate aminotransferase, alanine aminotransferase, alkaline phosphatase, and bilirubin in rats fed with the extracts. The protective effect could be attributed to the high contents of phenolics, most specifically iso-quercetin and quercetin. Different models of antioxidative stress have been used to study the antioxidant activity of coriander extracts *in vivo*. The aqueous and ethanolic extracts of coriander were investigated for their antioxidant properties in lead nitrate-induced hepatotoxicity in mice. As expected, treatment with lead nitrate (40 mg/kg) caused toxicity in the liver with an increased level of TBARS and a decrease in SOD and CAT activity and glutathione content.

Administration of coriander extracts (250–600 mg/kg) attenuated the effect of lead nitrate as shown by an increase in antioxidant content and activity. Histological examination revealed that at high doses, coriander extracts were able to restore the liver and kidney tissue to their normal structures as compared to tissue damage observed in the lead nitrate without extract supplementation. Although the study concluded that coriander extracts do prevent or slow down oxidative damage caused by lead, there is still a need to identify the specific metabolite and mechanism of action involved [56].

Coriander extracts, rich in phenolics and carotenoids, were fed to Wistar rats for 30 and 60 days. Initially, the aqueous extract was more effective, but towards the end of the study, the ether extract was found to be more effective in both liver and plasma as assessed by measuring TBARS levels [57]. Free radicals and lipid peroxidation have also been implicated in acute gastric lesions. The aqueous suspension of coriander seeds showed dose-dependent protection against gastric ulcers induced by various agents such as sodium chloride, sodium hydroxide, ethanol, and indomethacin as well as by pylorus ligation accumulated gastric acid secretion. The protective effect against ulcers was attributed to the free radical scavenging capacity of antioxidants in the seeds and the hydrophobic interactions of antioxidant compounds to form protective layers [58]. In a contradictory study published recently, essential oil from coriander seeds showed pro-oxidant activity both *In vitro* and *in vivo*.

Although the essential oil was shown to have some DPPH radical scavenging activity (IC50 4.05 mL/mL), it enhanced oxidation in lipid peroxidation with poor hepatoprotective effect in CCl_4-induced hepatotoxicity. Pretreatment with coriander oil resulted in decreased CAT activity and glutathione content [59]. This is partially supported by Wangensteen *et al.* [50], who reported that coriander oil and lipophilic extracts failed to show antioxidant properties in the *in vivo* study. In light of the above-reviewed evidence, it is clear that different parts of coriander do show some antioxidant activity *In vitro*, but there are contradictory reports concerning its effect in the *in vivo* models. Therefore, more studies are needed to elucidate the effect of coriander extract on the oxidation status of the body, especially, under *in vivo* conditions.

Anti-diabetic Activity

Diabetes is one of the most prevalent and rapidly growing diseases [60]. As there is no cure for diabetes, the patients have to take chemical drugs life-long, exposing them to the multiple side-effects of these drugs. This has compelled the scientists to search for more effective and safer anti-diabetic treatments. Coriander is traditionally used as a remedy against diabetes [61]. In several countries, including Saudi Arabia and Morocco, coriander seeds are still used as antidiabetic treatment [19, 62]. Several scientific studies have revealed the anti-hyperglycemic potential of coriander seeds [62 - 65]. Intake of coriander seed supplemented diet (62.5 g/kg) or drinking water mixed with seed decoction (2.5 g/L) decreased hyperglycemia in streptozotocin-induced diabetic mice. In a sub-chronic 30 day study, the aqueous extract of coriander seeds administered as a single dose per day (20 mg/kg) reduced plasma glucose and restored the normoglycemic state in obese-hyperglycemic-hyperlipidemic rats [66]. The treatment also reduced insulin resistance, total cholesterol, low-density lipoproteins (LDL)-cholesterol and triglycerides. These effects of coriander extract were found to be comparable to that of glibenclamide. Mechanistic studies involving *In vitro* and *in vivo* models revealed that the anti-hyperglycemic effect of coriander seeds is mediated through an increase in glucose uptake, glucose metabolism, and a dose-dependent increase in insulin secretion. The antihyperglycemic effect in the animal model was evident at a dose of 200 and 250 mg/kg of ethanolic extract of seeds [65, 67]. In another study, pretreatment with coriander seed powder caused changes in the carbohydrate metabolism; increased concentration of hepatic glycogen and activity of glycogen synthase [64]. Therefore, decreased glycogenolysis and gluconeogenesis and enhanced activities of glucose-6-phosphate dehydrogenase along with other glycolytic enzymes might all be an indication of the antihyperglycemic activity of coriander seeds. Consequently, they considered coriander as a potential source of useful dietary supplements for improving blood glucose control and preventing long-term complications in type 2 diabetes mellitus [49, 68, 69].

Conversely, the effect of administration of coriander essential oil on diabetes in experimental animals is not well studied. Nevertheless, the hypoglycemic activity of coriander essential oil compounds namely linalool, geranyl acetate, and γ-terpinene have been ascertained and the presence of this synergistic combination could be contributed to the hypoglycemic action of coriander essential oil [70].

Antihyperlipidemic Activity

Concerning its traditional medicinal uses, numerous studies have been carried out to investigate the effect of administration of coriander seeds on different aspects of lipid metabolism in experimental animals [71, 72].

In a 30 days sub-chronic study, oral administration of the aqueous extract of coriander seeds to obese hyperlipidemic rats reduced total cholesterol, LDL cholesterol, and triglycerides levels [73]. Furthermore, the administration of coriander seed oil to the rats fed with high cholesterol diet decreased the serum levels of total lipids (TLs), total cholesterol, triacylglycerols, and LDL-cholesterol. Pure coriander seed oil proved more effective in anti-hypercholesterolemic effect as compared to a mix of oils containing coriander oil [74]. The activity of HMG-CoA reductase, a key enzyme in cholesterol biosynthesis, was also decreased. The lipid-lowering effect was attributed to enhanced hepatic degradation of cholesterol and increased hepatic and fecal bile acids concentration. Dhanapakiam *et al.* [72] further confirmed the anti-cholesterolemic effect of coriander in their study and reported a general decrease in cholesterol and triglyceride levels in rats treated with coriander supplementation. A reduction in LDL and VLDL levels was also observed, suggesting a decrease in the activity of HMG CoA reductase. The supplementation also caused an increase in HDL cholesterol alongside accelerating the activities of lecithin cholesterol acyltransferase. The observed increase in the concentration of hepatic and fecal bile acids and steryl esters was again suggestive of the enhanced hepatic clearance of cholesterol. More recently, coriander was reported to transactivate the transcription factor and peroxisome proliferator-activated receptors that may improve overall lipid profile [75].

Health Effects on the Central Nervous System

In Iranian traditional medicine, coriander has been used for its anticonvulsant, anti-depressant, nerve soothing, sedative, and anxiolytic properties for ages. These activities have been validated by numerous scientific reports. The anti-epileptic potential of coriander seeds has been assessed using Pentylene Tetrazole (PTZ) and maximal electroshock test. The aqueous and ethanolic extracts of the coriander seeds tested in this study showed anticonvulsant activity manifested as delayed onset of clonic convulsion in the PTZ test and a decrease in the duration of tonic seizures in the maximal electroshock test [76]. The effect was comparable to phenobarbital at the dose of 5 mg/kg. These findings were confirmed by another report, whereby; aqueous-alcoholic extract of coriander and its essential oil caused dose-dependent protection against PTZ-induced tonic convulsions and death. The extract was found more effective than essential oil in increasing the onset time for myoclonic and clonic seizures [77].

In another study, the same extract and the essential oil (100–600 mg/kg) were assessed on mice for their sedative activity. The aqueous extracts at 200, 400, and 600 mg/kg doses prolonged pentobarbital-induced sleeping time than the control group, whereas, the essential oil showed a sedative effect only at 600 mg/kg, suggesting that the sedative constituents of coriander seeds might have been isolated in higher amount in the polar solvent [78]. To explore a natural and safer alternative to benzodiazepines, the anxiolytic effect of coriander seeds extract (100 mg/kg) was studied in mice, using the elevated plus-maze model [79]. The effect was recorded as a percentage of the time spent by mice in the open arms of the plus-maze and was found comparable to diazepam (0.3mg/kg). In this study, the coriander extract (50–500 mg/kg) also exhibited a sedative effect and demonstrated muscle relaxant potential manifested as reduced spontaneous activity and improved neuromuscular coordination, in a dose-dependent manner. In a later study, the anxiolytic effect of coriander seed extract was more comprehensively evaluated by Mahendra and Bisht [80] using multiple anxiety models in mice, such as elevated plus-maze test, open field test, light and dark test, and social interaction test. The aqueous-alcoholic extract of coriander seed (100 and 200 mg/kg) exhibited anxiolytic effect comparable with that of a standard drug, diazepam (0.5 mg/kg).

Furthermore, the aqueous extract of coriander seed was studied for its effect on anxiety and pain [81] using elevated plus-maze and hot plate models for anxiety and pain, respectively. At a dose of 200 mg/kg, the aqueous extract showed an anxiolytic effect comparable to the standard drug, diazepam (0.3 mg/kg). It also exhibited analgesic activity with an EC_{50} value of 200 mg/kg.

The aqueous extract and fixed oil from coriander seed have also shown anti-depressant activity in the experimental studies. The activity was assessed as the effect on the 'Immobility Time' of mice in forced swimming and tail suspension tests. The aqueous and diethyl ether extracts of coriander seeds have also shown significant anti-depressant like activity in the clinical settings. The activity was found comparable to fluoxetine and imipramine, commonly used anti-depressant drugs. The diethyl ether extract showed better efficacy as compared to its aqueous counterpart. The antidepressant activity was found as mediated through the inhibition of MAO-B activity, an enzyme implicated in the pathogenesis of depression [82]. A relatively recent study revealed the potential of fresh coriander leaves supplementation to reverse memory deficits [83]. The effect was determined against age-induced memory deficits in the aged animals and scopolamine and diazepam induced amnesia in the young animals and was measured as transfer latency using the elevated plus-maze model. Coriander leaves supplementation for 45 days successfully reversed the memory deficits in the old animals and the induced amnesia in the young animals. The activity was found as mediated through inhibition of ACE activity in the brain of both old and young animals and reduced serum cholesterol levels. The results of the study also suggested possible neuroprotective effects of the coriander leaves.

Anti-mutagenic Activity

A majority of cancer patients rely on natural product extracts as complementary and alternative medicine the world over [84].

Scientific studies have demonstrated anti-mutagenic activity in coriander. The compounds, aromatic amines, have the potential to be transformed into mutagens both in humans and animals. The aqueous crude coriander juice significantly decreased the mutagenicity of metabolized aromatic amines as assessed by using the Ames reversion mutagenicity assay (his- to his+) with the *Salmonella typhimurium* strain as an indicator organism. The anti-mutagenic effect was found to be positively correlated with chlorophyll content of the juice [85]. In another study, the effect of coriander extract was assessed on the murine neuroblastoma cell line (Neuro-21 cells). The murine neuroblastoma cell line is established from a spontaneous tumor and is considered a good tumor model. However, in this study, coriander extract was shown to have a weak anti-tumor effect, with an LC_{50} value of more than 5 mg/mL. Cell viability was assessed by the resazurin (Almar Blue) indicator assay [86].

Diuretic and Anti-hypertensive Activities

The traditional use of coriander as a diuretic agent for hypertension or to treat renal disorders has been reported in many cultures [87, 88]. In a study, the extract of coriander seeds was evaluated for its diuretic effect in anesthetized rats. The results showed that intravenous infusion of coriander seed extract caused a dose-dependent increase in urine output accompanied by an increase in the excretion of electrolytes and glomerular filtration rate, similar to that of the standard drug, furosemide [89].

The aqueous-methanolic extract of coriander seeds was also found to exhibit a diuretic effect in conscious rats [90]. The coriander extract also caused a blood pressure-lowering effect in anesthetized rats. *In vitro* testing showed the presence of vasodilator effect in the extract which was mediated through a combination of endothelial-dependent (cholinergic) and independent (Ca^{++} channel blockade) pathways [90].

Analgesic and Anti-inflammatory Effect

Non-steroidal Anti-inflammatory Drugs (NSAIDs) are commonly used to relieve pain and inflammation but are not free from the undesirable effects particularly gastrointestinal tract irritation [91]. Similarly, their COX-2 selective counterparts, although considered less ulcerogenic, have been reported to cause fatal cardiac toxicity. Therefore, there is an increasing need for safer anti-inflammatory drugs.

Several studies have shown that plant-derived bioactive constituents, such as flavonoids and dietary polyphenols, possess an anti-inflammatory effect involving various molecular targets [92, 93]. The anti-inflammatory effect of coriander seed is evident from its being one of the principal components of traditional Sri Lankan formulation; Maharasnadhi Quather (MRQ). Both animal and human studies have shown anti-inflammatory properties in MRQ. Administration of MRQ significantly inhibited carrageenan-induced rat paw edema. The formulation also increases pain tolerance in rats by 57% after 1 h of treatment as assessed by the hot plate test. The analgesic effect was suggested to be mediated *via* a supra-spinal effect. Supplementation of MRQ in patients suffering from rheumatoid arthritis for 3 months improved pain, inflammation, and mobility without any adverse effects on liver functions and gastrointestinal activities [94]. A poly-herbal formulation, consisting of coriander as one of the constituents, showed an inhibitory effect against inflammatory bowel disease. The activity was comparable to that of prednisolone [95].

The topical anti-inflammatory effect of lipolotion formulation supplemented with 0.5% and 1% of the coriander oil was tested on human volunteers for the anti-inflammatory effect. The formulation effectively reduced the UV-induced erythema in all the 40 volunteers though it was less effective than hydrocortisone. Coriander oil also showed a mild anti-inflammatory effect without causing any undesirable topical effects at both the concentrations tested [96].

In addition, the aqueous extract of coriander seed was studied for its effect on pain using a hot plate model [81]. The extract showed an analgesic effect with a median effective dose of 200 mg/kg. Among the isolated plant constituents, it has been reported that linalool, a monoterpene alcohol, found as a major component of coriander essential oil, plays a major role in the analgesic activity [97]. In this context, some workers reported the antinociceptive activity of linalool [98] while others studied the contribution of the glutamatergic system in the antinociception elicited by linalool in mice [99].

Digestive Activities

As a component of numerous indigenous herbal formulations, coriander is used to relieve several gastrointestinal ailments including dysentery, flatulence, vomiting, and indigestion. The digestive and carminative role of coriander has been shown due to increased secretion of bile with high bile acid content. Likewise, it also enhances the activities of both intestinal and pancreatic digestive enzymes. These stimulatory actions accelerate the overall digestion and reduce the food transit time in the gastrointestinal tract [100].

SAFETY STUDIES ON CORIANDER SEEDS

The safety profile of coriander has been assessed by a few studies. The coriander oil was tested on male and female rats for 28 days at the doses of 160, 400, and 1000 mg/kg. The resultant toxicities appeared as dose and gender-dependent. The high doses of coriander oil caused an increase in the weights of the liver and kidney in both male and female rats. The effect was accompanied by an increase in the total protein and albumin levels which were evident in female rats at medium/high doses and male rats at the high doses only. There was an increase in serum calcium levels in the male rats administered with 1000 mg/kg coriander oil and a high incidence of degenerative lesions in the renal cortex. Whereas, the hepatocellular changes including hepatocellular cytoplasmic vacuolization were more prominent in females. The reproductive organs were unaffected in both sexes. This study concluded that the non-observed effect level for males was 160 mg/kg, and for females, it should be less than 160 mg/kg [101].

The plant is traditionally used as an antifertility agent in Saudi Arabia. In a study, the reproductive toxicity of the aqueous extract of fresh coriander seeds was assessed on male and female rats. Oral administration of the extract at 250 mg and 500 mg/kg doses decreased implantation dose-dependently, possibly due to decreased progesterone levels; however, complete infertility was not observed. There was no effect on the weight of the fetuses and deformities were not observed [20]. In another investigation to assess the endocrinal and reproductive effects of coriander, its administration (250 mg/kg for 7 days) did not cause any histopathological changes in the tissues of male rabbits as compared to the control group. The testosterone secreting cells were found active, with no significant differences in testosterone production. The serum chemistry profile of both treated and untreated animals was comparable. The cholesterol levels of the treated group also remained unchanged [102].

Studies on the mutagenicity of coriander reported conflicting results. Ethanolic extract of coriander seeds failed to show any mutagenicity in rat embryo fibroblasts as studied with the Comet assay [103]. Contrary to this, Coriander juice was proven to be anti-mutagenic in action [104]. Linalool, the principal component of coriander essential oil, was found antimutagenic at 25 mg/mL, and it did not cause any chromosomal alterations in the Chinese hamster fibroblast assay [105] and unscheduled DNA synthesis in rat hepatocytes [106]. However, a couple of studies reported the mutagenicity of coriander. In a study reported by Mahmoud *et al.* [107], coriander fruit extract showed mutagenic activity in the Ames assay consisting of *Salmonella typhimurium* strains (TA98 and TA100). In a later study, the aqueous extract of coriander leaves at high concentrations (8 mg/mL) was associated with mutagenicity in two additional strains of *Salmonella typhimurium* (TA97/TA102), as assessed by Ames test. The same concentration also induced apoptosis and necrosis in human cell lines (WRL-68 and 293Q) and altered cell cycle [108].

The topical application of coriander oil and its components has generally been found safe. There is sufficient evidence to suggest that the essential oil does not irritate the skin. Application of coriander essential oil and linalool in 48 h closed patch test did not produce irritation in human subjects [109, 110]. There was no irritation associated with the application of 20% linalool in both healthy volunteers and patients suffering from skin problems [111].

CONCLUDING REMARKS

Different parts of coriander have been traditionally used for culinary and a range of medicinal purposes across various civilizations. The plant is also widely used as a food supplement in Asia and the Middle East due to the presence of beneficial constituents including petroselinic acid in seed oil and linalool in the essential oil. Scientific investigations revealing multiple biological activities including antioxidant, anti-mutagenic, antimicrobial, sedatives, anxiolytic, anti-depressant, neuro-protective, anti-diabetic, diuretic, anti-hypertensive, lead-detoxifying, and gut modulatory effects, have made the plant popular in other parts of the word too. Coriander has been validated as a safe source of valuable health-promoting constituents, although the essential oil and fixed oil of this plant are not sufficiently explored for their health benefits. Based on the safety and efficacy profile of the plant, it can be concluded that the medicinal use of coriander at the usual dosage is safe for human consumption as a food ingredient and in cosmetics.

CONSENT FOR PUBLICATION

Not applicable.

CONFLICT OF INTEREST

The authors declare that there is no conflict of interest in this chapter.

ACKNOWLEDGEMENTS

Declared none.

REFERENCES

[1]   Bhat S, Kaushal P, Kaur M, Sharma HK. Coriander (*Coriandrum sativum* L.): processing, nutritional and functional aspects. Afr J Plant Sci 2014; 8: 25-33.
[http://dx.doi.org/10.5897/AJPS2013.1118]

[2]   Duke JA, Bogenschutz-Godwin MJ, Pu Celliar J, Duke PAK. Handbook of medicinal herbs. 2nd ed. Boca Raton: CRC Press 2002; p. 222.
[http://dx.doi.org/10.1201/9781420040463]

[3]   Diederichsen A. Rugayah. *Coriandrum sativum* L. In: de Guzman CC, Siemonsma JS, Eds. Plant Resources of South-East Asia (PROSEA) No 13: Spices. Leiden: Backhuys Publisher 1999; pp. 104-8.

[4]   van Harten AM. Coriander: the history of an old crop. Landbouwkd Tijdschr 1974; 86: 58-64. [in Dutch].

[5]   Diederichsen A. Coriander (Coriandrum sativum L) Promoting the conservation and use of underutilized and neglected crops 3. Rome: Institute of Plant Genetics and Crop Plant Research, Gatersleben/ International Plant Genetic Resources Institute 1996.

[6]   Li H. The vegetables of ancient China. Econ Bot 1969; 23: 253-60.
        [http://dx.doi.org/10.1007/BF02860457]

[7]   Ceska O, Chaudary SK, Warrington P, Ashwood-Smith MJ, Bushnell GW, Poulton GA. Coriandrin, a novel, highly photoactive compound isolated from *Coriandrum sativum*. Phytochemistry 1988; 27: 2083-7.
        [http://dx.doi.org/10.1016/0031-9422(88)80101-8]

[8]   Diederichsen A. Coriander- Coriandrum sativum L Promoting the conservation and use of underutilized and neglected plants. IPGRI Videlle Sotte Chiese 1996.

[9]   Coskuner Y, Karababa E. Physical properties of coriander seeds (*Coriandrum sativum* L.). J Food Engin 2007; 80: 408-16.

[10]   Handa SS, Kaul MK. Supplement to Cultivation and Utilization of Medicinal Plants. Jammu Tawi: CSIR 1996; pp. 54-5.

[11]   Jamuna P, Rao PN, Reddy PV, Rao MR. Phosphorus requirement of coriander in black clay soil of low available P2O5. Indian Cocoa Arecanut Spices J 1991; 14: 112-3.

[12]   Gil A, De La Fuente EB, Lenardis AE, *et al.* Coriander essential oil composition from two genotypes grown in different environmental conditions. J Agric Food Chem 2002; 50(10): 2870-7.
        [http://dx.doi.org/10.1021/jf011128i] [PMID: 11982413]

[13]   Verma A, Pandeya SN, Yadav SK, Singh S, Soni P. A review on *Coriandrum sativum* (Linn.): an ayurvedic medicinal herb of happiness. J Adv Pharm Healthc Res 2011; 1: 28-48.

[14]   Varier PS. Coriandrum sativum in Indian medicinal plants: a compendium of 500 species (2). Chennai: Orient Longman LtD 1994; pp. 416-7.

[15]   Khan SW, Khatoon S. Ethnobotanical studies on some useful herbs of Haramosh and Bugrote valleys in Gilgit, northern areas of Pakistan. Pak J Bot 2008; 40: 43-58.

[16]   Ugulu I, Baslar S, Yorek N, Dogan Y. The investigation and quantitative ethnobotanical evaluation of medicinal plants used around Izmir province, Turkey. J Med Plants Res 2009; 3: 345-67.

[17]   Leung AY, Foster S. Encyclopedia of common natural ingredients used in food, drugs and cosmetics. 2nd ed., New York: John Wileys & Sons 1996.

[18]   Kapoor LD. Handbook of Ayurvedic Plants. Florida: CRC Press 1990; p. 44.

[19]   Al-Rowais NA. Herbal medicine in the treatment of diabetes mellitus. Saudi Med J 2002; 23(11): 1327-31.
        [PMID: 12506289]

[20]   Otoom SA, Al-Safi SA, Kerem ZK, Alkofahi A. The use of medicinal herbs by diabetic Jordanian patients. J Herb Pharmacother 2006; 6(2): 31-41.
        [http://dx.doi.org/10.1080/J157v06n02_03] [PMID: 17182483]

[21]   Bnouham M, Mekhfi H, Legssyer A, Ziyyat A. Ethnopharmacology Forum Medicinal plants used in the treatment of diabetes in Morocco. Int J Diabetes Metab 2002; 10(1): 33-50.
        [http://dx.doi.org/10.1016/j.jep.2006.09.011] [PMID: 17052873]

[22]   Eddouks M, Maghrani M, Lemhadri A, Ouahidi ML, Jouad H. Ethnopharmacological survey of medicinal plants used for the treatment of diabetes mellitus, hypertension and cardiac diseases in the south-east region of Morocco (Tafilalet). J Ethnopharmacol 2002; 82(2-3): 97-103.
        [http://dx.doi.org/10.1016/S0378-8741(02)00164-2] [PMID: 12241983]

[23]   Abu-Rabia A. Herbs as a food and medicine source in Palestine. Asian Pac J Cancer Prev 2005; 6(3): 404-7.

[PMID: 16236008]

[24]   Al-Said MS, Al-Khamis KI, Islam MW, Parmar NS, Tariq M, Ageel AM. Post-coital antifertility activity of the seeds of *Coriandrum sativum* in rats. J Ethnopharmacol 1987; 21(2): 165-73. [http://dx.doi.org/10.1016/0378-8741(87)90126-7] [PMID: 3437767]

[25]   Msaada K, Hosni K, Ben Taarit M, Hammami M, Marzouk B. Effects of growing region and maturity stages on oil yield and fatty acid composition of coriander (*Coriandrum sativum* L.) fruit. Sci Hortic (Amsterdam) 2009; 120: 525-31. [http://dx.doi.org/10.1016/j.scienta.2008.11.033]

[26]   Sriti J, Wannes WA, Talou T, Mhamdi B, Cerny M, Marzouk B. Lipid profile of Tunisian coriander (*Coriandrum sativum*) seed. J Am Chem Soc 2010; 87: 395-400.

[27]   Sriti J, Talou T, Wannes WA, Cerny M, Marzouk B. Essential oil, fatty acid and sterol composition of Tunisian coriander fruit different parts. J Sci Food Agric 2009; 89: 1659-64. [http://dx.doi.org/10.1002/jsfa.3637]

[28]   Ramadan MF, Mörsel JT. Oil composition of coriander (*Coriandrum sativum* L.) fruitseeds. Eur Food Res Technol 2002; 215: 2045-9. [http://dx.doi.org/10.1007/s00217-002-0537-7]

[29]   Sriti J. WannesWA, Talou T, Mhamdi B, Handaoui G, Marzouk B. Lipid fatty acid and tocol distribution of coriander fruits' different parts. Ind Crops Prod 2010; 31: 294-300. [http://dx.doi.org/10.1016/j.indcrop.2009.11.006]

[30]   Burt S. Essential oils: their antibacterial properties and potential applications in foods-a review. Int J Food Microbiol 2004; 94(3): 223-53. [http://dx.doi.org/10.1016/j.ijfoodmicro.2004.03.022] [PMID: 15246235]

[31]   Anwar F, Sulman M, Hussain AI, Saari N, Iqbal C, Rashid U. Physicochemical composition of hydro-distilled essential oil from coriander (*Coriandrum sativum* L.) seeds cultivated in Pakistan. J Med Plants Res 2011; 5: 3537-44.

[32]   Zheljazkov VD, Pickett KM, Caldwell CD, Pincock JA, Roberts JC, Mapplebeck L. Cultivar and sowing date effects on seed yield and oil composition of coriander in Atlantic Canada. Ind Crops Prod 2008; 28: 88-94. [http://dx.doi.org/10.1016/j.indcrop.2008.01.011]

[33]   Telci I. TO G, Sahbaz N. Yield, essential oil content and composition of *Coriandrum sativum* varieties (var. vulgare Alef and var. microcarpum DC.) grown in two different locations. J Essent Oil Res 2006; 18: 189-93. [http://dx.doi.org/10.1080/10412905.2006.9699063]

[34]   Singh G, Maurya S, de Lampasona MP, Vega M, Catalan CA. Studies on essential oils, Part 41. Chemical composition, antifungal, antioxidant and sprout suppressant activities of coriander (*Coriandrum sativum*) essential oil and its oleoresin Flavour fragr J 2006; 21: 472-9.

[35]   Bhuiyan MNI, Begum J, Sultana M. Chemical composition of leaf and seed essential oil of *Coriandrum sativum* L. from Bangladesh. Bangladesh J Pharmacol 2009; 4: 150-3. [http://dx.doi.org/10.3329/bjp.v4i2.2800]

[36]   de Figueiredo RO, Nakagawa J, Ming LC, Marques MOM. Composition of Coriander Essential Oil from Brazil. XXVI International Horticultural Congress: The Future for Medicinal and Aromatic Plants. 692.

[37]   Msaada K, Hosni K, Taarit MB, Chahed T, Kchouk ME, Marzouk B. Changes on essential oil composition of coriander (*Coriandrum sativum* L.) fruits during three stages of maturity. Food Chem 2007; 102: 1131-4. [http://dx.doi.org/10.1016/j.foodchem.2006.06.046]

[38]   Zoubiri S, Baaliouamer A. Essential oil composition of Coriandrumsativum seed cultivated in Algeria as food grains protectant. Food Chem 2010; 122: 1226-8.

[http://dx.doi.org/10.1016/j.foodchem.2010.03.119]

[39] Nejad Ebrahimi S, Hadian J, Ranjbar H. Essential oil compositions of different accessions of *Coriandrum sativum* L. from Iran. Nat Prod Res 2010; 24(14): 1287-94.
[http://dx.doi.org/10.1080/14786410903132316] [PMID: 20803372]

[40] Barros L, Dueňas M, Dias MI, Sousa MJ, Santos-Buelga C, Ferreira ICFR. Phenolic profiles of *in vivo* and *In vitro* grown *Coriandrum sativum* L. Food Chem 2012; 132: 841-8.
[http://dx.doi.org/10.1016/j.foodchem.2011.11.048]

[41] Kandlakunta B, Rajendran A, Thingnganing L. Carotene content of some common (cereals, pulses, vegetables, spices and condiments) and unconventional sources of plant origin. Food Chem 2008; 106: 85-9.
[http://dx.doi.org/10.1016/j.foodchem.2007.05.071]

[42] Kitajima J, Ishikawa T, Fujimatu E, Kondho K, Takayanagi T. Glycosides of 2-C-methyl-D-erythritol from the fruits of anise, coriander and cumin. Phytochemistry 2003; 62(1): 115-20.
[http://dx.doi.org/10.1016/S0031-9422(02)00438-7] [PMID: 12475627]

[43] Kubo I, Fujita K, Kubo A, Nihei K, Ogura T. Antibacterial activity of coriander volatile compounds against Salmonella choleraesuis. J Agric Food Chem 2004; 52(11): 3329-32.
[http://dx.doi.org/10.1021/jf0354186] [PMID: 15161192]

[44] Saeed S, Tariq P. Antimicrobial activities of Emblica officinalis and *Coriandrum sativum* against Gram-positive bacteria and Candida albicans. Pak J Bot 2007; 39: 913-7.

[45] Matasyoh JC, Maiyo ZC, Ngure RM, Chepkorir R. Chemical composition and antimicrobial activity of essential oil of *Coriandrum sativum*. Food Chem 2009; 113: 526-9.
[http://dx.doi.org/10.1016/j.foodchem.2008.07.097]

[46] Begnami AF, Duarte MCT, Furletti RV. Antimicrobial potential of *Coriandrum sativum* L. against different candida species *In vitro*. Food Chem 2010; 118: 74-7.
[http://dx.doi.org/10.1016/j.foodchem.2009.04.089]

[47] Lo Cantore P, Iacobellis NS, De Marco A, Capasso F, Senatore F. Antibacterial activity of *Coriandrum sativum* L. and *Foeniculum vulgare* Miller Var. vulgare (Miller) essential oils. J Agric Food Chem 2004; 52(26): 7862-6.
[http://dx.doi.org/10.1021/jf0493122] [PMID: 15612768]

[48] Chaudhry NM, Tariq P. Bactericidal activity of black pepper, bay leaf, aniseed and coriander against oral isolates. Pak J Pharm Sci 2006; 19(3): 214-8.
[PMID: 16935829]

[49] Chithra V, Leelamma S. Hypolipidemic effect of coriander seeds (*Coriandrum sativum*): mechanism of action. Plant Foods Hum Nutr 1997; 51(2): 167-72.
[http://dx.doi.org/10.1023/A:1007975430328] [PMID: 9527351]

[50] Wangensteen H, Samuelson AB, Malterud KE. Antioxidant activity in extracts of coriander. Food Chem 2004; 88: 293-7.
[http://dx.doi.org/10.1016/j.foodchem.2004.01.047]

[51] Ramadan MF, Kroh LW, Mörsel JT. Radical scavenging activity of black cumin (*Nigella sativa* L.), coriander (*Coriandrum sativum* L.), and niger (*Guizotia abyssinica* Cass.) crude seed oils and oil fractions. J Agric Food Chem 2003; 51(24): 6961-9.
[http://dx.doi.org/10.1021/jf0346713] [PMID: 14611155]

[52] Ramadan MF, Wahdan KMM. Blending of corn oil with black cumin (Nigella sativa) and coriander (*Coriandrum sativum*) seeds oil: impact on functionality, stability and radical scavenging activity. Food Chem 2012; 132: 873-9.
[http://dx.doi.org/10.1016/j.foodchem.2011.11.054]

[53] Ramadan MF. Healthy blends of high linoleic sunflower oil with selected cold pressed oils: functionality, stability and antioxidative characteristics. Ind Crops Prod 2013; 43: 65-72.

[http://dx.doi.org/10.1016/j.indcrop.2012.07.013]

[54]   Hashim MS, Ling S, Remya R, Teena M, Anila L. Effect of polyphenolic compounds from *Coriandrum sativum* on H_2O_2-induced oxidative stress in human lymphocytes. Food Chem 2005; 92: 653-60.
[http://dx.doi.org/10.1016/j.foodchem.2004.08.027]

[55]   Pandey A, Bigoniya P, Raj V, Patel KK. Pharmacological screening of *Coriandrum sativum* Linn. for hepatoprotective activity. J Pharm Bioallied Sci 2011; 3(3): 435-41.
[http://dx.doi.org/10.4103/0975-7406.84462] [PMID: 21966166]

[56]   Kansar L, Sharma V, Sharma A, Lodi S, Sharma SH. Protective role of coriandrum sativum(coriander) extracts against lead nitrate induced oxidative stress and tissue damage in malemice. Int J Appl Biol Pharm Technol 2011; 2: 65-83.

[57]   Melo EA, Bion IM, Filho JM, Guerra NB. *In vivo* antioxidant effect of aqueous and etheric coriander (*Coriandrum sativum* L.) extracts. Eur J Lipid Sci Technol 2003; 105: 483-7.
[http://dx.doi.org/10.1002/ejlt.200300811]

[58]   Al-Mofleh IA, Alhaider AA, Mossa JS, Al-Sohaibani MO, Rafatullah S, Qureshi S. Protection of gastric mucosal damage by *Coriandrum sativum* L. pretreatment in Wistar albino rats. Environ Toxicol Pharmacol 2006; 22(1): 64-9.
[http://dx.doi.org/10.1016/j.etap.2005.12.002] [PMID: 21783688]

[59]   Samojlik I, Lakić N, Mimica-Dukić N, Daković-Svajcer K, Bozin B. Antioxidant and hepatoprotective potential of essential oils of coriander (*Coriandrum sativum* L.) and caraway (*Carum carvi* L.) (Apiaceae). J Agric Food Chem 2010; 58(15): 8848-53.
[http://dx.doi.org/10.1021/jf101645n] [PMID: 20608729]

[60]   Wild S, Roglic G, Green A, Sicree R, King H. Global prevalence of diabetes: estimates for the year 2000 and projections for 2030. Diabetes Care 2004; 27(5): 1047-53.
[http://dx.doi.org/10.2337/diacare.27.5.1047] [PMID: 15111519]

[61]   Lewis WH. Elvin-LewisMPF Medical Botany: Plants Affecting Man's Health. New York: Wiley 1977.

[62]   Tahraoui A, El-Hilaly J, Israili ZH, Lyoussi B. Ethnopharmacological survey of plants used in the traditional treatment of hypertension and diabetes in south-eastern Morocco (Errachidia province). J Ethnopharmacol 2007; 110(1): 105-17.
[http://dx.doi.org/10.1016/j.jep.2006.09.011] [PMID: 17052873]

[63]   Swanston-Flatt SK, Day C, Bailey CJ, Flatt PR. Traditional plant treatments for diabetes. Studies in normal and streptozotocin diabetic mice. Diabetologia 1990; 33(8): 462-4.
[http://dx.doi.org/10.1007/BF00405106] [PMID: 2210118]

[64]   Chithra V, Leelamma S. *Coriandrum sativum*- mechanism of hypoglycemic action. Food Chem 1999; 67: 229-31.
[http://dx.doi.org/10.1016/S0308-8146(99)00113-2]

[65]   Eidi M, Eidi A, Saeidi A, *et al.* Effect of coriander seed (*Coriandrum sativum* L.) ethanol extract on insulin release from pancreatic beta cells in streptozotocin-induced diabetic rats. Phytother Res 2009; 23(3): 404-6.
[http://dx.doi.org/10.1002/ptr.2642] [PMID: 19003941]

[66]   Gray AM, Flatt PR. Insulin-releasing and insulin-like activity of the traditional anti-diabetic plant *Coriandrum sativum* (coriander). Br J Nutr 1999; 81(3): 203-9.
[http://dx.doi.org/10.1017/S0007114599000392] [PMID: 10434846]

[67]   Aissaoui A, El-Hilaly J, Israili ZH, Lyoussi B. Acute diuretic effect of continuous intravenous infusion of an aqueous extract of *Coriandrum sativum* L. in anesthetized rats. J Ethnopharmacol 2008; 115(1): 89-95.
[http://dx.doi.org/10.1016/j.jep.2007.09.007] [PMID: 17961943]

[68]   Gallagher AM, Flatt PR, Duffy G, Abdel-Wahab YHA. The effects of traditional antidiabetic plants on *In vitro* glucose diffusion. Nutr Res 2003; 23: 413-24.
[http://dx.doi.org/10.1016/S0271-5317(02)00533-X]

[69]   Pandeya KB, Tripathi IP, Mishra MK, *et al.* A critical review on traditional herbal drugs: an emerging alternative drug for diabetes. Int J Org Chem (Irvine) 2013; 3: 1-22.
[http://dx.doi.org/10.4236/ijoc.2013.31001]

[70]   Abou El-Soud NH, El-Lithy NA, El-Saeed GSM, *et al.* Efficacy of C*oriandrum Sativum* L. essential oil as antidiabetic. J Appl Sci Res 2012; 8: 3646-55.

[71]   Lal AA, Kumar T, Murthy PB, Pillai KS. Hypolipidemic effect of *Coriandrum sativum* L. in triton-induced hyperlipidemic rats. Indian J Exp Biol 2004; 42(9): 909-12.
[PMID: 15462185]

[72]   Dhanapakiam P, Joseph JM, Ramaswamy VK, Moorthi M, Kumar AS. The cholesterol lowering property of coriander seeds (*Coriandrum sativum*): mechanism of action. J Environ Biol 2008; 29(1): 53-6.
[PMID: 18831331]

[73]   Aissaoui A, Zizi S, Israili ZH, Lyoussi B. Hypoglycemic and hypolipidemic effects of *Coriandrum sativum* L. in Meriones shawi rats. J Ethnopharmacol 2011; 137(1): 652-61.
[http://dx.doi.org/10.1016/j.jep.2011.06.019] [PMID: 21718774]

[74]   Ramadan MF, Amer MMA, Awad AE. Coriander (*Coriandrum sativum* L.) seed oil improves plasma lipid profile in rats fed a diet containing cholesterol. Eur Food Res Technol 2008; 227: 1173-82.
[http://dx.doi.org/10.1007/s00217-008-0833-y]

[75]   Mueller M, Beck V, Jungbauer A. PPARα activation by culinary herbs and spices. Planta Med 2011; 77(5): 497-504.
[http://dx.doi.org/10.1055/s-0030-1250435] [PMID: 20957597]

[76]   Hosseinzadeh H, Madanifard M. Anticonvulsant effect of *Coriandrum sativum* L. seed extract in mice. Arch Iran Med 2000; 3: 81-4.

[77]   Ghoreyshi E, Ghazal HM. Effect of extract and essential oil of *Coriandrum sativum* seed against pentylenetetrazole induced seizure. J Pharm Sci 2008; 3: 1-10.

[78]   Ghoreyshi E, Hamedani H. Sedative-hypnotic activity of extracts of essential oil of coriander seeds. Int J Mol Sci 2006; 31: 22-7.

[79]   Emamghoreishi M, Khasaki M, Aazam MF. *Coriandrum sativum*: evaluation of its anxiolytic effect in the elevated plus-maze. J Ethnopharmacol 2005; 96(3): 365-70.
[http://dx.doi.org/10.1016/j.jep.2004.06.022] [PMID: 15619553]

[80]   Mahendra P, Bisht S. Anti-anxiety activity of *Coriandrum sativum* assessed using different experimental anxiety models. Indian J Pharmacol 2011; 43(5): 574-7.
[http://dx.doi.org/10.4103/0253-7613.84975] [PMID: 22022003]

[81]   Pathan AR, Kothawade KA, Logade MN. Anxiolytic and analgesic effect of seeds of *Coriandrum sativum*Linn. Int J Res Pharm Chem 2011; 1: 1087-99.

[82]   Kharade SM, Gumate DS, Patil VM, Kokane SP, Narikwade NS. Behavioral and biochemical studies of seeds of *Coriandrum sativum* in various stress models of depression. Int J Curr Res Rev 2011; 1003: 4-8.

[83]   Mani V, Parle M, Ramasamy K, Abdul Majeed AB. Reversal of memory deficits by *Coriandrum sativum* leaves in mice. J Sci Food Agric 2011; 91(1): 186-92.
[http://dx.doi.org/10.1002/jsfa.4171] [PMID: 20848667]

[84]   Yates JS, Mustian KM, Morrow GR, *et al.* Prevalence of complementary and alternative medicine use in cancer patients during treatment. Support Care Cancer 2005; 13(10): 806-11.
[http://dx.doi.org/10.1007/s00520-004-0770-7] [PMID: 15711946]

[85]   Cortés-Eslava J, Gómez-Arroyo S, Villalobos-Pietrini R, Espinosa-Aguirre JJ. Antimutagenicity of coriander (*Coriandrum sativum*) juice on the mutagenesis produced by plant metabolites of aromatic amines. Toxicol Lett 2004; 153(2): 283-92.
[http://dx.doi.org/10.1016/j.toxlet.2004.05.011] [PMID: 15451560]

[86]   Mazzio EA, Soliman KF. *In vitro* screening for the tumoricidal properties of international medicinal herbs. Phytother Res 2009; 23(3): 385-98.
[http://dx.doi.org/10.1002/ptr.2636] [PMID: 18844256]

[87]   Grieve M. Coriander a modern herbal: the medicinal, culinary, cosmetic and economic properties, cultivation and folk-lore. New York: Dover Publications 1971.

[88]   Eddouks M, Maghrani M, Lemhadri A, Ouahidi ML, Jouad H. Ethnopharmacological survey of medicinal plants used for the treatment of diabetes mellitus, hypertension and cardiac diseases in the south-east region of Morocco (Tafilalet). J Ethnopharmacol 2002; 82(2-3): 97-103.
[http://dx.doi.org/10.1016/S0378-8741(02)00164-2] [PMID: 12241983]

[89]   Aissaoui A, Zizi S, Israili ZH, Lyoussi B. Hypoglycemic and hypolipidemic effects of *Coriandrum sativum* L. in Meriones shawi rats. J Ethnopharmacol 2011; 137(1): 652-61.
[http://dx.doi.org/10.1016/j.jep.2011.06.019] [PMID: 21718774]

[90]   Jabeen Q, Bashir S, Lyoussi B, Gilani AH. Coriander fruit exhibits gut modulatory, blood pressure lowering and diuretic activities. J Ethnopharmacol 2009; 122(1): 123-30.
[http://dx.doi.org/10.1016/j.jep.2008.12.016] [PMID: 19146935]

[91]   Graham DY, Agrawal NM, Roth SH. Prevention of NSAID-induced gastric ulcer with misoprostol: multicentre, double-blind, placebo-controlled trial. Lancet 1988; 2(8623): 1277-80.
[http://dx.doi.org/10.1016/S0140-6736(88)92892-9] [PMID: 2904006]

[92]   Yoon JH, Baek SJ. Molecular targets of dietary polyphenols with anti-inflammatory properties. Yonsei Med J 2005; 46(5): 585-96.
[http://dx.doi.org/10.3349/ymj.2005.46.5.585] [PMID: 16259055]

[93]   García-Lafuente A, Guillamón E, Villares A, Rostagno MA, Martínez JA. Flavonoids as anti-inflammatory agents: implications in cancer and cardiovascular disease. Inflamm Res 2009; 58(9): 537-52.
[http://dx.doi.org/10.1007/s00011-009-0037-3] [PMID: 19381780]

[94]   Thabrew MI, Dharmasiri MG, Senaratne L. Anti-inflammatory and analgesic activity in the polyherbal formulation Maharasnadhi Quathar. J Ethnopharmacol 2003; 85(2-3): 261-7.
[http://dx.doi.org/10.1016/S0378-8741(03)00016-3] [PMID: 12639750]

[95]   Jagtap AG, Shirke SS, Phadke AS. Effect of polyherbal formulation on experimental models of inflammatory bowel diseases. J Ethnopharmacol 2004; 90(2-3): 195-204.
[http://dx.doi.org/10.1016/j.jep.2003.09.042] [PMID: 15013181]

[96]   Reuter J, Huyke C, Casetti F, *et al.* Anti-inflammatory potential of a lipolotion containing coriander oil in the ultraviolet erythema test. J Dtsch Dermatol Ges 2008; 6(10): 847-51.
[http://dx.doi.org/10.1111/j.1610-0387.2008.06704.x] [PMID: 18371049]

[97]   Guimarães AG, Quintans JSS, Quintans LJ Jr. Monoterpenes with analgesic activity - a systematic review. Phytother Res 2013; 27(1): 1-15.
[http://dx.doi.org/10.1002/ptr.4686] [PMID: 23296806]

[98]   Peana AT, D'Aquila PS, Chessa ML, Moretti MDL, Serra G, Pippia P. (-)-Linalool produces antinociception in two experimental models of pain. Eur J Pharmacol 2003; 460(1): 37-41.
[http://dx.doi.org/10.1016/S0014-2999(02)02856-X] [PMID: 12535857]

[99]   Batista PA, Werner MFP, Oliveira EC, *et al.* Evidence for the involvement of ionotropic glutamatergic receptors on the antinociceptive effect of (-)-linalool in mice. Neurosci Lett 2008; 440(3): 299-303.
[http://dx.doi.org/10.1016/j.neulet.2008.05.092] [PMID: 18579302]

[100] Platel K, Srinivasan K. Digestive stimulant action of spices: a myth or reality? Indian J Med Res 2004; 119(5): 167-79.
[PMID: 15218978]

[101] Letizia CS, Cocchiara J, Lalko J, Api AM. Fragrance material review on linalool. Food Chem Toxicol 2003; 41(7): 943-64.
[http://dx.doi.org/10.1016/S0278-6915(03)00015-2] [PMID: 12804650]

[102] Al Suhaimi EA. Effect of *Coriandrum sativum*, a common herbal medicine on endocrine and reproductive organ structure and function. Internet J Alt Med 2009; 7.
[http://dx.doi.org/10.5580/3b1]

[103] Heibatullah K, Marzieh P, Arefeh I, Ebrahim M. Genotoxicity determinations of coriander drops and extract of *Coriandrum sativum* in cultured fibroblast of rat embryo by comet assay. Saudi Pharm J 2008; 16: 85-8.

[104] Cortes-Eslara J, Gomez-Arroyo S, Villalobos-Pietrini R. Espinosa- Aguire JJ. Antimutagenicity of coriander (*Coriandrum sativum*) juice on themetagenesis produced by plant metabolite of aromatic amines. Toxicol Lett 2004; 153: 283-92.
[http://dx.doi.org/10.1016/j.toxlet.2004.05.011] [PMID: 15451560]

[105] Ishidate M Jr, Sofuni T, Yoshikawa K, *et al.* Primary mutagenicity screening of food additives currently used in Japan. Food Chem Toxicol 1984; 22(8): 623-36.
[http://dx.doi.org/10.1016/0278-6915(84)90271-0] [PMID: 6381265]

[106] Heck JD, Vollmuth TA, Cifone MA, Jagannath DR, Myhr B, Curren RD. An evaluation of food flavoring ingredients in a genetic toxicity screening battery. Toxicologist 1989; 1: 257-68.

[107] Mahmoud I, Alkofahi A, Abdelaziz A. Mutagenic and toxic activities of several spices and some Jordanian medicinal plants. Int J Pharmacol 1992; 30: 81-5.

[108] Reyes MR, Reyes-Esparza J, Angeles OT, Rodríguez-Fragoso L. Mutagenicity and safety evaluation of water extract of Coriander sativum leaves. J Food Sci 2010; 75(1): T6-T12.
[http://dx.doi.org/10.1111/j.1750-3841.2009.01403.x] [PMID: 20492211]

[109] Kligman AM. Report to Research Institute for Fragrance Materials (RIFM) . 1970.

[110] Kligman AM. Report to Research Institute for Fragrance Materials (RIFM) . 1971.

[111] Fuji T, Furukawa S, Suzuki S. Compounded perfumes for toilet goods-non irritative compounded perfumes for soaps. Yukagaku 1972; 21: 904-8.

CHAPTER 4

The Fenugreek Seed: Therapeutic Properties and Applications

Sana Riaz, Muhammad A. Hafeez and **Abid A. Maan**[*]

National Institute of Food Science and Technology, University of Agriculture, Faisalabad, Pakistan

Abstract: Fenugreek (*Trigonella foenum-graecum*), belonging to the family Leguminosae, is a distinctive therapeutic plant. Several parts of the plant (leaves, roots and seeds) are used as a spice, food, culinary herb, and in traditional medicines. It has been frequently referred in Ayurveda for its various health benefits. Fenugreek seeds contain high phytonutrients, minerals, and vitamin contents. They have high amount of non-starch polysaccharide (NSP) fibers. Major NSP's are tannins, saponins, hemicelluloses, mucilages and galactomannans. Non-starch polysaccharides enhance bowel movement, support in smooth digestion and also help in decreasing LDL-cholesterol level in the blood through binding. NSPs also capture toxic substances present in food and act as a shield for the colon mucosal layers against cancers. Fenugreek seeds also contain amino acid 4-hydroxyisoleucine, which boosts insulin secretion. Other essential phytochemicals present in fenugreek seeds (including trigonelline, gitogenin, yamogenin diosgenincholine and trigogenin) play important therapeutic roles, such as being anti-anorexic, anti-oxidant, anti-carcinogenic, anti-hyperlipidemic, anti-inflammatory, and antidiabetic uses, *etc*. The present chapter discusses various biological and therapeutic properties and uses of fenugreek in detail, along with its toxicological considerations.

Keywords: 4-hydroxyisoleucine, Anti-diabetic, Cardio-protective, Fenugreek seed powder, Fenugreek seed, Galactomannan, Hyperlipidemia, Saponins, *Trigonella foenum graecum* L, Trigonelline.

INTRODUCTION

Fenugreek (biologically recognized as *Trigonella foenum-graecum* L.) belongs to the family Leguminosae. It is an annual dicotyledonous crop having white flowers, branched stems, yellow seeds, trifoliate leaves, and roots having nodules (see Fig. **1**) [1, 2]. It is basically cultivated as a wild crop in Mediterranean areas of West Asia and South-Eastern Europe. India is considered as the second largest

---
[*] **Corresponding author Abid A. Maan:** National Institute of Food Science and Technology, University of Agriculture, Faisalabad, Pakistan; Tel: 03324516417, 041-9200161; E-mail: abid.maan@uaf.edu.pk

Atta-ur-Rahman, M. Iqbal Choudhary & Sammer Yousuf

origin of fenugreek, where it is recognized as an ancient crop of the region [3, 4].

Carbonized fenugreek seed was discovered from Rohilla village of Punjab (India), demonstrating its trade and use by Harappan civilization (2000-1700 BC). The utilization of fenugreek and its seeds as a spice and to preserve mummies has been reported in ancient Egypt. Seeds and leaves are mostly used for spicing and flavoring in many dishes due to their strong aroma and flavor [5]. Application of fenugreek as "green manure" crop has also been documented because of its ability to produce high biomass in less period of time, thus enhancing the level of organic matter in the soil [6].

Fenugreek plant comprises branches and sub-branches having light green or light yellow to white leaves on either auxiliary or terminal position. The plant differs in height from 15 to 45 cm, with dry land crops shorter in height than irrigated plants. The plant produces copious single long pods of 10 to 15 cm having 17 to 20 seeds (on average). Sometimes double pods are also found under natural field conditions [3, 7]. The pods are long and curved, having short hair on the surface. The younger pods are green to light purple and become brown at maturity [8, 9]. Chemical and physical mutagenesis of the plant has resulted in bulk production of double pods as well as an increased number of seeds per plant [7]. Seeds vary from round to rectangular shape, and are green in color when immature. At maturity, the seeds become solid, hard and brown [1, 10]. Fenugreek is slightly sweet and pleasantly bitter in taste. The seeds (whether ground or whole) are utilized in many dishes for flavor [11].

Other applications of fenugreek, documented in the literature, include its use as hey, silage, swath or straight grazing, water reservation and fixation of nitrogen from the environment into the soil [12 - 15]. The current focus of the most fenugreek breeding programs is to produce good quality seed (fast-maturing, disease-resistant and high yielding verities) for specific climatic conditions [16].

Composition of Fenugreek Seeds

The seeds contain 44-58% carbohydrates (specially galactomannans), 6-11% lipids (especially the unsaturated fatty acids), and 20-30% proteins (rich in arginine, glycine and alanine while deficient in methionine and lysine). The major free amino acid present in seeds is 4-hydroxyisoleucine. As compared to other legumes, fenugreek seeds contain a high amount of minerals (Fe, P, Zn, Ca, Mn, and P). The seeds also contain trigonelline (a fundamental alkaloidal constituent) and some aromatic components, including nonalactone, n-alkanes and sesquiterpenes. Three steroidal saponins, namely diosgenin, tigogenin and gitogenin, are also found in fenugreek seeds [17 - 19]. A comprehensive summary of various components found in fenugreek seeds is presented in Table **1** [3, 20].

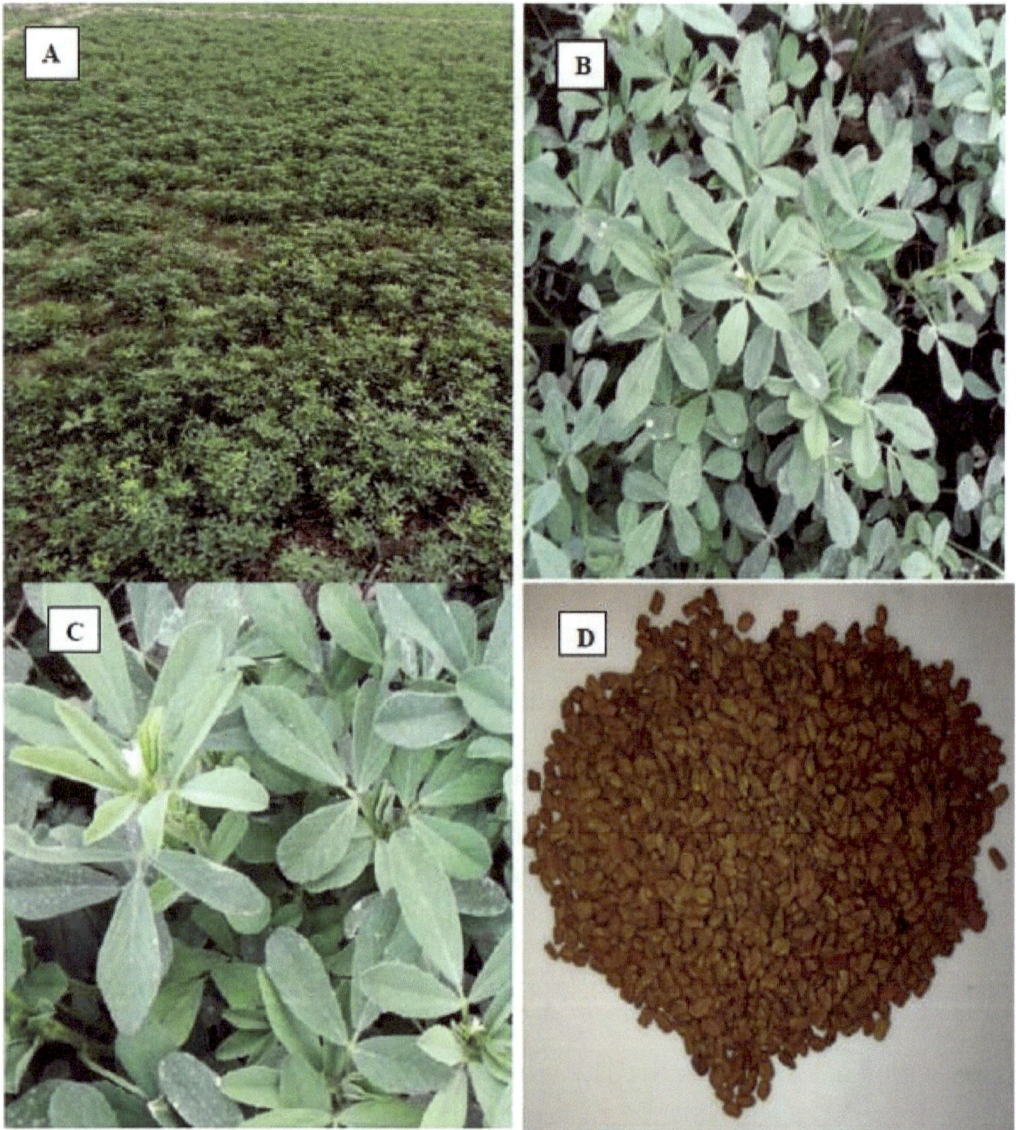

Fig. (1). A typical representation of (A) Fenugreek crop (B) Fenugreek leaves (C) Fenugreek flower and (D) Fenugreek seeds.

Table 1. Chemical constituents of fenugreek seeds.

Amino acids	Tryptophan, 4-hydroxyisoleucine, arginine, histidine, lysine, threonine, valine and methionine
Alkaloids	Carpaine, trigonelline, gentianine and choline
Flavonoids	Apigenin, luteolin, quercetin, kaempferol, naringenin, myricetin, tricin and catechin

(Table 1) cont.....

Saponins	Diosgenin, tigogenin and gitogenin
Lipids	Phospholipids, glycolipids, oleic acid, linoleic acid and linolenic acid,
Carbohydrates	Galactomannans, soluble and insoluble fibers
Minerals	Iron, zinc, calcium, phosphorous and manganese

Galactomannans

Galactomannans (GAL) are the members of seed gums, which are chemically heterogeneous polysaccharides composed of β-(1–4)-d-mannan with one d-galactose branch linked α-(1–6) (see Fig. **2**) [21]. These gums are found in the endosperm of dicotyledonous seeds of many plants, specially Leguminosae. There are 4 basic origins of seed galactomannans *i.e.* tara (*Caesalpinia spinosa* Kuntze), guar (*Cyamopsis tetragonoloba*), locust bean (*Ceratonia siliqua*), and fenugreek. These galactomannans contain variable ratios of galactose and mannose (G:M) as well as the distribution of galactopyranosyl molecules within mannan chains [22, 23]. The difference in galactose distribution and composition with mannan main chain are responsible for changes in rheology, solubility and viscosity in relation to other polymers. The viscosity and solubility increase when G:M ratio increases from 1:4 (in lotus bean gum) to 1:3 (in tara gum) and 1:2 (in guar gum). Fenugreek galactomannans have a G:M ratio of 1:1 which makes them superior regarding their gel-forming properties, as compared to other galactomannans [24 - 26].

It has been reported that galactomannan fibers slow down the absorption of carbohydrates by enhancing the viscosity of digesta in the gut. This affects the postprandial plasma glucose response. Moreover, they have also been reported to have an anti-diabetic effect by enhancing the production of GLP-1 in the intestine [27, 28]. Anti-diabetic properties of GLP-1 (including inhibition of glucagon production, stimulation of insulin secretion and slow gastric emptying) have been reported in several studies [29]. Furthermore, GLP-1 has been reported to reduce systolic blood pressure with an improved lipid profile when consumed as supplements. Fenugreek seeds, being a rich source of galactomannan fibers (around 28%), can be used in clinical diets recommended for diabetic patients [30].

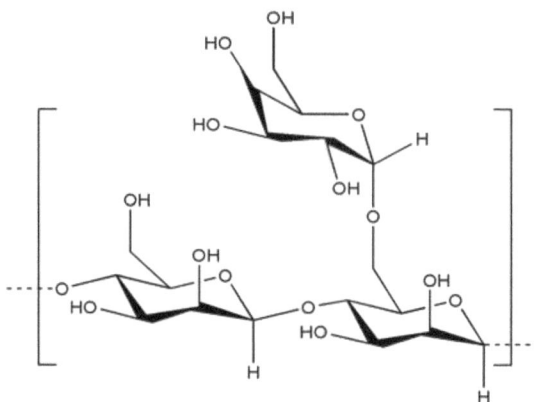

Fig. (2). Chemical structure of galactomannan.

Saponins

Saponins are amphiphilic compounds comprising polar saccharide chains (uronic acid, pentose or hexose) combined with non-polar aglycones. The saccharide chains contain one or more linear oligosaccharides having a chain length of 2-5 sugar molecules. The d-glucose, d-xylose, d-glucuronic acid, l-rhamnose, l-arabinose and d-galactose are common sugars of saccharide chain. Saponins contain polycyclic rings (30 carbon triterpene or 27 carbon sterol) in their aglycone units. The Asian fenugreek seeds have steroidal saponins primarily in the form of diosgenin, tigogenin, and gitogenin (see Fig. **3**). Sugar molecules are linked at one or two glycosylation sites to aglycones through glycosidic linkages [31, 32]. The bitter part of saponins is hydrophobic while the sugar part is hydrophilic. These structures of saponins provide characteristic surface properties to make oil-in-water emulsions as well as to serve as defensive colloids. In addition, they enables the saponins to tightly bound to other components of the plant [33].

Saponins (extracted from fenugreek seeds) have exhibited hypocholesterolemic effects in several *in vivo* and *In vitro* investigations through binding of bile acids [34, 35]. They restrict the reabsorption of bile salts in gut and thus fasten the breakdown of cholesterols. Saponins have also been reported to exhibit antioxidant properties. Such a property is seen to be strongly associated with the soybean derived saponins; however, the antioxidant potential of saponins derived from fenugreek seeds has not been characterized yet [36].

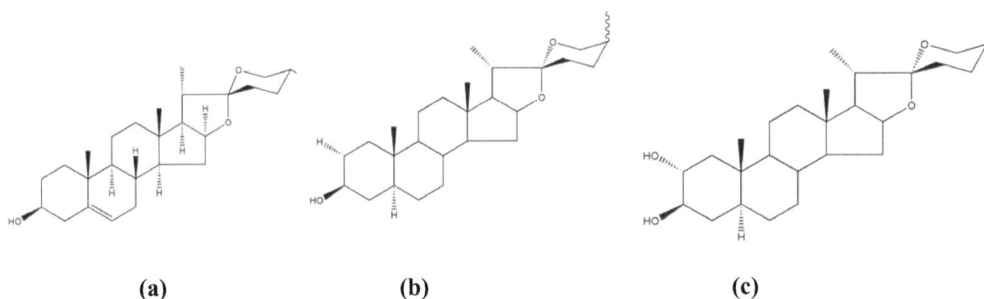

Fig. (3). Chemical structures of different forms of steroidal saponins (a) diosgenin, (b) tigogenin, and (c) gitogenin.

4-Hydroxyisoleucine (4-OH-Ile)

4-OH-Ile is a polar non-charged branched-chain amino acid (see Fig. **4**) abundantly found in fenugreek seeds (0.015%-0.4%). It is synthesized from isoleucine and has been hypothesized as a molecule responsible for the antidiabetic potential in animals due to its pancreatic insulin secretion regulating capacity [37]. 4-OH-Ile accounts for almost 80% of the total free amino acids in fenugreek seeds [38]. Ogawa, Kodera [39] investigated the effect of OH-Ile in obese mice fed at HFD and recommended that OH-Ile can be considered as an effective anti-obesity compound. 4-OH-Ile also reported as blood glucose level, lowering agent improves liver functions, and minimize lipotoxicity [40].

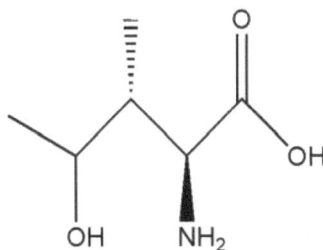

Fig. (4). Chemical structure of 4-Hydroxyisoleucine (4-OH-Ile).

Trigonelline

Trigonelline ($C_7H_7NO_2$) is a plant hormone that regulates plant growth and survival. It is an alkaloid mainly found in oats, coffee beans, hemp seeds, fenugreek seeds and garden peas. It is named as "trigonelline" because it was first derived from fenugreek seeds. It is a methylated form of vitamin B_3 (niacin) and hence also named as methylated niacin. At a high temperature, it breaks down to niacin. Trigonelline acts as an amino acid due to the presence of quaternary ammonium group with carboxylate, and thus exists as zwitterion (see Fig. **5**).

Trigonelline has been reported to have many therapeutic effects, including anticarcinogenic, hypocholesterolemic and anti-diabetic effect [3, 41 - 43].

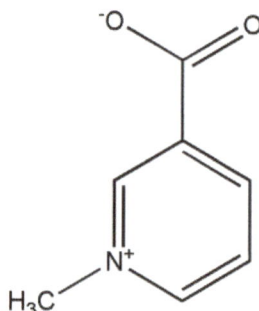

Fig. (5). Chemical structure of trigonelline.

BIOLOGICAL POTENTIAL OF FENUGREEK SEEDS

The biological potential of fenugreek seeds, in terms of antifungal and antibacterial activities, has been reported by several studies and is summarized in Table **2**.

Anti-fungal Activity

Fungi affect most of the crops before harvesting or during storage under unfavorable conditions. Some fungi produce phytotoxins which affect sprout growth on the surface of seeds and germination of seeds while some others produce mycotoxins that affect quality of food [44]. Fenugreek seeds contain defensins and defensin-like proteins that shield seeds from soil fungi and hence increase survival rate of seedlings. Such defensins extracted from seeds can be used for various antifungal applications. Tf_AFP having molecular weight of 10.3 kDa extracted from fenugreek seeds has been reported to exhibit the antifungal activity against several fungal species including *Rhizoctonia solani, Fusarium solani*, and *Fusarium oxysporum* [45]. The antifungal activity of seed oil tested against *Aspergillus niger* has been reported to result in complete inhibition (100%) of fungal activity [46]. Similar effects have also been reported by other studies in literature [44, 47 - 49].

Anti-bacterial Activity

The antibacterial activity of fenugreek seeds has been well documented in literature. The aqueous extracts of seeds have exhibited antimicrobial activity against a wide range of bacterial strains. Among tested strains *E. coli*, and

Staphylococcus aureus were found to be most susceptible; whereas *Shigella flexeneri* and *Salmonella enterica* were reported to be the most resistant [50].

Walli, Al-Musrati [51] investigated the antimicrobial potential of aqueous (boiling, hot and cold) and methanolic extracts of fenugreek seeds against a number of gram positive and gram negative bacteria including *Escherichia coli* (*E. coli*), *Staphylococcus epidermis* (*St. epidermis*), *Proteus vulgaris* (*P. vulgaris*), *Candida albicans* (*C. albicans*), *Staphylococcus saprophyticus* (*St. saprophyticus*), and *Staphylococcus aureus* (*St. aureus*). Only the boiling water extracts showed antimicrobial activity while both methanol and cold water extracts could not inhibit microbial activity. Sulieman, Ahmed [46] investigated the inhibitory potential of fenugreek seed oil against three bacterial species (*Staphylococcus aureus, Escherichia coli*, and *Salmonella typhimurium*) and reported that seed oil has a strong antimicrobial activity against all tested microorganisms. Other studies reporting antimicrobial activity of seeds include [47, 52 - 57].

Table 2. Summary of biological effects of fenugreek seeds.

Active Compound/Preparation	Effect	Reference
Antifungal		
Antifungal peptide (Tf_AFP)	Inhibited the growth of many fungal species such as *Rhizoctonia solani, Fusarium solani*, and *Fusarium oxysporum*	[45]
Seed oil	Retard growth of human pathogens *i.e.* Aspergillus fumigatus and *Aspergillus niger*	[47]
Seed extract	Inhibit growth of *Penicillium italicum* (25-32%).	[58]
Antibacterial		
Aqueous extracts	Inhibited the growth of many microbial strains such as *E. coli* and *Staphylococcus aureus*	[50]
Seed oil	Inhibitory potential against *Staphylococcus aureus, Escherichia coli* and *Salmonella typhimurium*) and one mould (*Aspergillus niger*)	[46]
Ethanol seed extract	Active against *Bacillus subtilis, E coli, L. bacillus, S. aureus, Vibrio cholerae, S. typhi* and *M. lutea*.	[55]
Seed oil	Active against *Klebsiella pneumoniae, Proteus, E coli, Pseudomonas aeruginosa* and *S. aureus*	[52]
Seed extract	The antibacterial activity against pathogenic Gram-negative (*S. typhi, Klebsiella pneumoniae, E coli, Pseudomonas aeruginosa*) and Gram-positive (*S. aureus*)	[59]

THERAPEUTIC POTENTIAL OF FENUGREEK SEEDS

Therapeutic potential of fenugreek seeds has been intensively investigated and several studies have reported their antioxidative, anti-inflammatory, anti-obesity, cardiovascular, hepatoprotective and other beneficial effects. These therapeutic effects have been discussed in detail in following sections, and are summarized in Table **3**.

Anti-oxidant activity

Antioxidants are the agents that scavenge free radicals and prevent or inhibit cell oxidation due to free radicals. Antioxidants are capable of neutralizing free radicals and reduce or prevent oxidative damages to lipid, enzymes, DNA, proteins carbohydrates *etc.* and reduce the risk of chronic diseases [60]. Principal sources of natural antioxidants are whole grains, vegetables and fruits. Natural antioxidants belong to several classes of compounds with a wide diversity of chemical and physical properties. Fenugreek seeds possess promising beneficial effects against oxidative stress that can be attributed to three major bioactive components *i.e.* diosgenin, 4-OH-Ile, and fibers [61 - 64].

Oxidative stress; characterized by higher generation of ROS, has been linked with etiology of various human diseases. Antioxidants have potential of neutralizing ROS and their activity is believed to be beneficial for preventing oxidative damage. Belguith-Hadriche, Bouaziz [65] evaluated the antioxidant potential (*in vivo* study) of different extracts (hexane, water, dichloro-methane, methanol, ethyl acetate) of fenugreek seeds. Oral administration of ethyl acetate extracts significantly lowered the level of SOD, TBARS and catalase in the liver, heart and kidneys of rats fed with high cholesterol diet.

In another (*In vitro*) study, fenugreek seed extract was reported to scavenge ABTS and DPPH radicals. The anti-mutagenic potential of the extract was reported following the inhibition of γ-radiation induced strand break formation in plasmid pBR322 DNA [66]. Furthermore, fenugreek seed intake resulted in a remarkable reduction in hs-CRP as compared to the control group while the anti-oxidant and anti-inflammatory activity of FSP was evaluated by human trials. Fenugreek seed significantly increases SOD activity while it does not impart significant changes in glutathione peroxidase activity, serum interleukin (IL)-6, and tumor necrosis factor-α [67].

Mukthambaand Srinivasan [68] investigated the cardio-protective effect of fenugreek seeds on experimentally induced myocardial infarction. As oxidation of LDL is major cause in the arteriosclerotic process, the potential of fenugreek in reduction of LDL oxidation has been observed in rats. It was recommended that under both normal conditions and hypercholesterolemic conditions dietary fenugreek is proved to be protective against LDL oxidation. Several other studies had also revealed antioxidant potential of fenugreek seed [69 - 71].

Anti-diabetic Activity

Diabetes mellitus (DM) is a major endocrine metabolic disorder described by increase in blood glucose level. This results from insulin production deficiency by endogenous insulin ineffectiveness or by pancreatic β-cells [29]. DM is one of the most widespread metabolic disorders worldwide with vast health, economic and social consequences. According to World Health Organization (WHO)'s forecasts, diabetes will be the 7th main cause of death in 2030. T2DM accounts for 90-95% of total cases resulting from insulin resistance which usually develops due to accumulation of secondary metabolites of lipids [67]. There are four different mechanisms with which fenugreek seeds reduce the blood glucose levels [41]:

- Inhibition of glucose absorption from gastrointestinal tract or intestine
- Effect on pancreas, employing an insulin secretagogue or insulin mimetic effect
- Increase in peripheral blood glucose absorption, normalization of select processes and enhance insulin receptor density
- Reduction of pro-inflammatory factors which reduce insulin resistance

Several studies support either secretagogue or insulin-mimetic effects of fenugreek on the pancreas in case of elevated blood glucose level or inhibition of absorption of glucose in the intestine. Low molecular weight galactomannans (isolated from fenugreek seeds) have exhibited anti-hyperglycemic against alloxan-induced hyperglycemia in rats [29]. Trigonelline is reported to reduce blood glucose level in mice as well as in humans by improving insulin level and enhancing insulin sensitivity. Antidiabetic and anti-dyslipidemic effect of trigonelline was studied on high-fat-fed diabetic rats. Supplementation of trigonelline reduced AST, ALP, glucose, ALT, glycosylated hemoglobin, cholesterol, triglycerides, free fatty acids levels and improved the muscle glycogen and hepatic insulin levels [72].

Robert, Ismail [73] evaluated the hyperglycemic effect of seed powder supplemented (10%) buns and flatbread on humans. It was concluded that every gram of seed powder can be considered to decrease 4.2% of food glycemic index. Jin, Shi [74] also demonstrated that fenugreek seeds prevent diabetic nephropathy development in a STZ-challenged diabetic rats. Singh, Tamarkar [75] evaluated the antihyperglycaemic and antidyslipidaemic properties of 4-OH-Ile in mice and recorded a significant decline in blood glucose, plasma insulin, TG, TC, LDL-C levels. Furthermore, some recent studies has also evaluated antidiabetic effect of fenugreek seed [76 - 78].

Anti-inflammatory

Inflammation is a process that contributes to pathologic events which cause damage in autoimmune diseases, tissue damage and inflammatory disorders [79]. Unrestrained neuro-inflammatory response is harmful to neurons and may cause disorders like Parkinson's disease, Alzheimer's disease and multiple sclerosis.

Trigonelline has been reported to lower hippocampal oxidative stress and inflammation in neuroinflammation induced rats [80]. Carrageenan-challenged paw edema mice were administered with methanolic extracts of fenugreek seeds. The anti-inflammatory and antinociceptive potentials of extracts were observed at a dose of 100 mg/kg that were attributed to alkaloids and flavonoids present in the extracts [81]. Cotton pellet-induced arthritic rats were treated with petroleum ether extract of fenugreek seeds and paw inflammation (in paw edema induced by formaldehyde and carrageenan) was reported to decrease up to 85%. In another study, a significant reduction of elevated SGPT and ALP activities in serum and liver of seed extract treated rats was observed by Pundarikakshudu *et al.*, Shah [82]. These findings evidence the strong anti-inflammatory potential of fenugreek seeds.

Anti-obesity

Obesity is currently indicated as global issue, and approximately all worldwide health organizations have explained its alarming occurrence. In 2017, report from Organization for Economic Co-operation and Development (OECD) demonstrated that overweight and obesity ratio were still accreting in many adults aged from 15-74 years. Regardless of their age, both young people and adults showed a raising trend in overall prevalence of obesity rates from year 1999 to year 2016, and this expansion is reported to be continuous [83]. Obesity is explained as the presence of excessive body fats as an adipose tissue and is basically caused by the chronic energy imbalances; where energy intake increases energy expenditure [84]. Obesity may progress to cancer, type-2 diabetes, respiratory disease, insulin resistance, coronary heart disease and osteoarthritis.

Seeds of fenugreek contain high contents of dietary fibers (48%). These dietary fibers (galactomannans) form a viscous gel in the human intestine and inhibit glucose and lipid absorption. Kumar, Bhandari [85] evaluated the inhibitory effect of aqueous seed extract on accretion of fat and dyslipidemia on HFD induced overweight rats. The treatment showed remarkable decrease in the gain in body weight, WAT weight, leptin, BMI, lipids, lipase, serum insulin, blood glucose and apolipoprotein-beta status. Ilavenil, Arasu [86] reported the role of trigonelline on inhibition of lipids accumulation and adipocyte differentiation in the 3T3-L1 cells. Treatment of adipocytes with the trigonelline down-regulates PPAR-γ mRNA and C/EBP-α expression which further down-regulate other genes like resistin, adiponectin, leptin, adipogenin and binding protein (aP2) of fatty acid adipocytes. The significant effects on expression of GLUT-4 and FAS in the trigonelline treated adipocytes were observed suggesting that the trigonelline inhibited adipogenesis by reducing the PPAR-γ-facilitated pathway during adipogenesis. Other studies providing the evidence of weight reduction and anti-obesity coupled with the diabetes and hyperlipidemia include [87, 88].

Anti-Cancer and Chemo-preventive Activity

Cancer is one of the leading health problems in the world and 2nd major cause of deaths in the United States [89]. Abasand Naguib [90] evaluated (*In vitro*) anticancer effects of germinated and dried seed extracts on pancreatic (AsPC-1) and human breast (MCF7) cells. Extracts of both germinated as well as dry seeds stimulated apoptosis in experimental cells; however, germinated seed extract showed greater potential as compared to dry seed extract. This difference can be attributed to the fact that germination enhances antioxidant components like trigonellin, tannins, phenolics, steroids, phytates, flavonoids and alkaloids; all possessing good anti-tumor activity. Shabbeer, Sobolewski [91] investigated the anticancer effect of fenugreek seed extract on prostate, pancreatic and breast cells and reported the inhibitory effect on these cells. The surprising outcome of this study was that cancer cells death occurred regardless of growth-stimulating pathways being concurrently upregulated by seed extracts.

Nuclear factor E2-related factor 2 is considered to have an important role in the development of cancer and chemo-resistance. Robert, Ismail [73] demonstrated that trigonelline caused efficient Nrf2 inhibition capable of blocking Nrf2-dependent proteasome activity, thereby stimulating apoptosis in pancreatic cancer cells. It was concluded that not only fenugreek seed extract but also active compounds (trigonelline and diosgenin) showed anticancer effects at the preclinical level.

Role in Cardiovascular Diseases

Cardiovascular disease (CVD) is a vast and linked pathologic term commonly known as cerebrovascular disease, congenital heart diseases, rheumatic, CHD, peripheral arterial disease, and venous thromboembolism. The risk factors of CVDs include diabetes, smoking, abdominal obesity, dyslipidemia, and hypertension. It accounts for 31% of mortality all around the world mostly in the form of congenital heart diseases and cerebrovascular accidents. Globally, CVD is not only the leading cause of deaths but also a leading cause of loss of disability-adjusted life years [92, 93]. WHO has recommended that early CVD is avoidable up to 75% and improvement in risk factors can help in decreasing its incidence. However, the development of CVD in advanced years is unavoidable; thus risk reduction is critical [92].

The effect of aqueous extract of fenugreek seeds on dyslipidemia and fat accumulation in HFD-induced obese rats was investigated [85]. The extract significantly increased adiponectin status and decreased blood glucose, BMI, lipids, body weight gain, WAT, serum insulin, apolipoprotein-B and leptin levels. Furthermore, it also improved lipid and glucose metabolism, elevated antioxidant protection, downregulated lipogenic enzymes and enhanced insulin sensitivity.

Sharma and Choudhary [94] investigated the influence of aqueous emulsified seed powder on rabbits with experimentally induced hyperlipidemia. The study revealed that seed powder significantly decreased the atherogenic index, serum TC, LDL-C and HDL-C in rabbits. However, no significant change was observed in VLDL-C and TG levels. Ramulu, Giridharan [95] studied the anti-hyperlipidemic potential of fenugreek seeds (10% and 20%) and galactomannan (2.5% and 5%) supplemented diets on the mutant obese rat strains (WNIN/GR-Ob). Lipid profile and body weight gain of rats was reduced significantly with no influence on their feed intake. Similarly, an increase in HMG-CoA reductase activity as well as a higher level of fecal neutral sterols excretion were observed. This links the hyperlipidemic effect of seed galactomannans with the increased activity of hepatic regulatory enzymes.

Role in Mental Health

Neuroinflammatory response, if uncontrolled, could be injurious to neurons and can cause diseases like Alzheimer's disease, multiple sclerosis and Parkinson's disease through activation and mobilization of various types of local cells within central nervous system involving astrocytes and microglia [80, 96]. Some changes occur in the immune system during aging that make the older people more susceptible to infections, including viral or bacterial infections [96]. Khalili, Alavi [80] investigated the beneficial effects of trigonelline against LPS-induced cognitive decline in rats. It reduced AChE activity and MDA whereas GSH, superoxide dismutase and catalase were increased. A dose-dependent pattern of trigonelline was reported to be better compared to some commercially-used drugs (dexamethasone). The LPS-challenged cognitive reduction was reduced by trigonelline through suppression of hippocampal oxidative stress, inflammation and suitable modulation of AChE and NF-κB/TLR4 activity. 4-OH-Ile is reported to produce an antidepressant effect in animal models of depression by brain serotonin turnover enhancement [97]. Makowska, Szczesny [98] and Khalil, Roshdy [99] have reported enhanced memory, increased learning and decreased neural cell deficits through fenugreek seeds. In addition, anti-Alzheimer's disease effects of fenugreek seeds have also been reported [100].

Hepatoprotective Potential

The liver is the largest gland and second largest organ of body after skin. Due to its vital and deliberate role, the liver is usually exposed to many external and internal materials such as drugs, viruses and chemical toxicants that could adversely affect the liver. Liver pathophysiology has been associated with various factors such as oxidative stress (difference in the production of reactive nitrogen and oxygen species RNS/ROS) and antioxidant contents in the body. RNS and ROS play a vital role in the induction and development of liver-related diseases while the non-enzymatic or enzymatic antioxidant system in the body offers defense against oxidative stress, which is mostly caused due to free radicals. It has been recognized that antioxidant-rich diet intake is inversely related with the risk of developing various liver diseases, signifying the role of focusing on natural antioxidants having low or no adverse effects for use in food and preventive medicine industry [101].

Effect of polysaccharides (extracted from fenugreek seeds) against insecticide-TMX-induced hepatotoxicity (in mice) was investigated by Feki, Jaballi [102]. A significant decrease in hematologic effects (caused by TMX injuries) was observed. Hepatoprotective role of a polyphenolic extract of seeds was evaluated in rats chronically administered with ethanol leading to liver dysfunction [103]. This resulted in cytochrome-b5 and cytochrome P450 activity stimulation and a decrease in phase II enzyme *i.e.* glutathione-S-transferase and cytochrome--reductase. Treatment with polyphenolic extract reestablished the markers level serving as a protective agent in the liver.

In rats with severe liver toxicity induced by aluminum chloride ($AlCl_3$) a liver protective effect was seen when rat diet was mixed with fenugreek seed powder resulting in (proximately) complete recovery based on histopathological and biochemical parameters [104].

Table 3. Summary of therapeutic effects of fenugreek seeds.

Active Compound/Preparation	Effect	Reference
Antioxidant		
Diosgenin and trigonelline	Beneficial effects in inflammation and oxidative stress	[61]

(Table 3) cont.....

Active Compound/Preparation	Effect	Reference
4-OH-Ile	Retardation of ROS generation, associated inflammation and restored insulin sensitivity	[63]
Seed powder	Reduced oxidation of serum LDL	[64]
Ethyl acetate extract	Reduced level of SOD, TBARS and catalase in liver, heart and kidney	[65]
FWEP	Significant recovery in oxidative parameters, compared to the TMX treated group	[102]
Anti-diabetic Activity		
Low molecular weight galactomannans	Anti-hyperglycemic potential against alloxan-induced hyperglycemia	[29]
Trigonelline	Reduced blood glucose levels, cholesterol, triglycerides and free fatty acids levels	[72]
Seed powder	Hyperglycemic effect on human	[73]
Anti-inflammatory		
Trigonelline	Suppression of hippocampal oxidative stress and neuroinflammation	[80]
Fractions of Methanolic extract	Alkaline chloroform fraction (antinociceptive effect) and Acidified chloroform fraction (anti-inflammatory effect) produced better effects	[81]
Anti-obesity		
Aqueous extract	remarkable decrease in the gain in body weight, white adipose tissue weight, leptin, BMI, lipids, lipase, serum insulin, blood glucose and apolipoprotein-beta status	[85]
Anti-cancer		
Aqueous extract of germinated and dry fenugreek seed	Significantly affected viability of breast and pancreatic cancer cells, DNA fragmentation, higher LDH levels, higher levels of caspase-3 & 6 and antioxidant effect	[90]
Seed extract	Cytotoxicity in prostatic, pancreatic and breast cells, cell cycle arrest in prostatic cells and inhibition prostatic cell growth	[91]
Trigonelline	Caused efficient Nrf2 inhibition capable of blocking Nrf2-dependent proteasome activity	[105]
Cardiovascular Disease		
Aqueous extract	Low levels of systolic, diastolic and arterial blood pressure	[85] .
Seed powder	Significant decrease in the atherogenic index, serum TC, LDL-C and HDL-C in Rabbits	[94]
Seed extract	Downregulate the fatty acid synthase, acetyl-CoA carboxylase and upregulate the peroxisome proliferator-activated receptor gamma	[106]

(Table 3) cont.....

Active Compound/Preparation	Effect	Reference
Role in Mental Health		
Trigonelline	Relieves lipopolysaccharide-induced learning and memory impairment	[80]
4-OH-Ile	Antidepressant effect	[97]
Saponins	Anti-Alzheimer effect	[99]
Fenugreek extract	Enhanced memory and decreased neural cell deficits associated with menopause	[100]
Hepatoprotective Potential		
Seed extract	Protective effect against insecticide- TMX-induced hepatotoxicity	[102]
Polyphenolic extract of seeds	Re-established the marker levels of liver damage and inverted changes in cytochrome-c reductase, alcohol-metabolizing, electron transport component and detoxification	[103]

CULINARY APPLICATIONS

Fenugreek seeds are carminative, aromatic, bitter, galactogouge and can be eaten raw and cooked. Major portion of the seed comprises of proteins and dietary fibers and have no flavor and taste [107]. Fenugreek paste prepared from ground seeds (traditionally known as Cemen) is a popular food in Turkey [108]. Fenugreek seeds are commonly used in stews, salads, soups, cauliflower, potato, beans and mango-based dishes in the Middle East countries and China. The ground seeds are the vital ingredient of oriental sauces, *halva* (a local sweet dish in India prepared from wheat semolina) and curry powders. Other culinary applications include in pickles, chutneys, confectionary, chewing gum, puddings, cakes, soft drinks, syrups (caramel, vanilla, maple and butterscotch) and ice creams [5]. The fiber-rich muffins prepared with fenugreek seed husk exhibited soft texture, good volume and medium fine grain [83]. Hegazyand Ibrahium [109] stated that the incorporation of germinated fenugreek seed flour (10%) in wheat biscuits enhanced their nutritional and chemical characteristics. Another study revealed that the incorporation of soaked (10%) and germinated (20%) fenugreek seed flour in wheat flour produced biscuits with good consumer acceptance and high nutritional value [110]. Waniand Kumar [111] have reported an improvement in quality characteristics of extruded snacks with fenugreek seeds incorporation. Similar effects of seed flour supplementation have been reported for quality and nutritional value of wheat and cornbread [112, 113]. The sprouted fenugreek seeds are reported to be used in sandwiches and salads. The seeds are also processed to make fenugreek tea and coffee which are consumed as soothing beverages in many parts of the world [114].

MISCELLANEOUS APPLICATIONS

Several studies have reported application of fenugreek seeds into cosmetics, animal feed *etc.* Akhtar, Waqas [13] have reported that emulsion formulation (cream) prepared form fenugreek seed extract exhibited significant enhancement properties including ageing, skin elasticity, fatigue and hydration of healthy human skin. Seed proteins and lecithin help to prevent hair loss; whereas, nicotinic acid enhances hair growth [115]. Noudeh, Sharififar [116] formulated shampoo from fenugreek seeds extract. The prepared shampoo exhibited excellent physicochemical properties including foam formation, wettability, viscosity, pH and conditioning.

Mamoun, Mukhtar [117] have reported that supplementation of fenugreek seeds in broiler feed can help to improve carcass characteristics resulting in high profits. Furthermore, its supplementation in goat feed results in increased milk yield and milk fats [107].

In foods, fenugreek seed extract has been employed as emulsifying, clarifying and thickening agent (owing to its galactomannan gums), while its essential oils have been used as an excellent natural preservative (owing to their antifungal, antibacterial and antioxidant properties) [118 - 120].

TOXICOLOGICAL CONSIDERATIONS

Several studies have reported toxicological effects of fenugreek, including reproductive, allergic, teratogenic, behavioral and neurophysiological [121 - 125]. Al-Yahya [122] investigated the effect of consumption of fenugreek seed (at high dosages of 305 and 610 mg/kg body weight) on the fertility of mice and reported enhanced number of DNA damaged abnormal sperms, reduced sperm amounts, reduced fertility and motility. In another study, the assessment of female rodents infertility demonstrated that oral intake of seeds (at the rate 200 mg/rat for 30 days) resulted in a remarkable reduction in hormone level, visible decline in ovary weight, increased number of inflammatory cells and significant dissolution of few [123]. Administration of aqueous seed extract to mice (100 and 500 mg/ kg body weight) resulted in teratogenic effects including increased pup death, growth inhibition, neurobehavior changes and malformations (development of bump and split palate on the head of newborns) during gestation in the post-weaning period [126]. Keeping in view the toxicological effects of fenugreek seeds, its excessive use continuously for an extended period of time should be avoided.

LIST OF ABBREVIATIONS

ABTS	2,2′-Azinobis 3-ethylbenzothiazoline-6-sulfonate
AChE	Acetylcholinesterase
ALT	Alanine transaminase
ALP	Alkaline phosphatase
AST	Aspartate Aminotransferase
BMI	Body mass index
CHD	Coronary heart disease
CVD	Cardiovascular disease
DM	Diabetes mellitus
DPPH	2,2′-diphenyl-1-picrylhydrazyl hydrate
FAS	Fatty acid synthase
FWEP	Fenugreek seed water polysaccharide
FSP	Fenugreek seed powder
GAL	Galactomannans
GLUT-4	Glucose transporter type 4
GLP-1	Glucagon-like peptide-1
GPX	Glutathione peroxidase
HDL	High density Lipoproteins
HFD	High-fat diet
4-OH-Ile	4-Hydroxyisoleucine
HMG-CoA	3-hydroxy-3-methyl-glutaryl-coenzyme A
hs-CRP	High-sensitivity C-reactive protein
IL	Serum interleukin
LDH	Lactate dehydrogenase
LDL	Low density lipoprotein
LPS	Lipopolysaccharide
Nrf2	Nuclear factor E2-related factor 2
PPAR-γ	Peroxisome proliferator-activated receptor
RNS	Reactive nitrogen species
ROS	Reactive oxygen species
SOD	Superoxide dismutase
STZ	Streptozotocin
TBARS	Thiobarbituric acid-reactive substances
TC	Total cholesterol

T2DM	Type 2 diabetes mellitus
TG	Triglyceride
Tf_AFP	Defensin-like antifungal peptide
TLR4	Trigonelline lowered toll-like
TMX	Thiamethoxam
VLDL	Very low-density lipoproteins

CONFLICT OF INTEREST

The authors declare no conflict of interest, financial or otherwise.

ACKNOWLEDGEMENTS

Declared none.

REFERENCES

[1]   Basu SK, Zandi P, Cetzal-Ix W. Chapter-28. Fenugreek (*Trigonella foenum-graecum* L.): Distribution, Genetic Diversity, and Potential to Serve as an Industrial Crop for the Global Pharmaceutical, Nutraceutical, and Functional Food Industries. The Role of Functional Food Security in Global Health Elsevier 2019; 471-97.
[http://dx.doi.org/10.1016/B978-0-12-813148-0.00028-1]

[2]   Sarwar S, Hanif MA, Ayub MA, Boakye YD, Agyare C. Chapter 20 - Fenugreek. In: Sarwar S, Nawaz H, Khan MM, Byrne HJ, Eds. Medicinal Plants of South Asia. Elsevier 2020; pp. 257-71.

[3]   Habtemariam S. The chemical and pharmacological basis of fenugreek (Trigonella foenum-graecum L.) as potential therapy for type 2 diabetes and associated diseases.Medicinal Foods as Potential Therapies for Type-2 Diabetes and Associated Diseases. Academic Press 2019; pp. 579-637.
[http://dx.doi.org/10.1016/B978-0-08-102922-0.00017-1]

[4]   Rahman MM, Ullah MO, Huq ME, Khan MW. Analysis of Fatty Acid Composition and Physicochemical Characteristic of *Trigonella foenum-graecum* Linn Ripe Seed by Gas Liquid Chromatography. MJ Chem 2019; 21(1): 24-8.

[5]   Kakani R, Anwer M. Handbook of herbs and spices. Elsevier 2012; pp. 286-98.

[6]   Acharya S, Thomas J, Basu S. Fenugreek: an "old world" crop for the "new world". Biodivers 2006; 7(3-4): 27-30.
[http://dx.doi.org/10.1080/14888386.2006.9712808]

[7]   Acharya S, Acharya K, Paul S, Basu S. Antioxidant and antileukemic properties of selected fenugreek (*Trigonella foenum-graecum* L.) genotypes grown in western Canada. Can J Plant Sci 2011; 91(1): 99-105.
[http://dx.doi.org/10.4141/cjps10025]

[8]   Solorio-Sánchez F, Solorio-Sánchez B, Basu S, *et al.* Opportunities to grow annual forage legume fenugreek (Trigonella foenum-graecum L) under mexican sylvopastoral system. Am J Social Issues Humanities 2014; pp. 86-95.

[9]   Basu S, Acharya S, Thomas J. A report on powdery mildew infestations caused by Erysiphe polygoni DC in North American grown fenugreek. J Mycopathol Res 2006; 44(2): 253-6.

[10]   Zandi P, Basu SK, Khatibani LB, Balogun MO, Aremu MO, Sharma M, *et al.* Fenugreek (*Trigonella foenum-graecum* L.) seed: a review of physiological and biochemical properties and their genetic

improvement. Acta Physiol Plant 2015; 37(1): 1714.
[http://dx.doi.org/10.1007/s11738-014-1714-6]

[11]   Şanlier N, Gencer F. Role of spices in the treatment of diabetes mellitus: A minireview. Trends Food Sci Technol 2020; 99: 441-9.
[http://dx.doi.org/10.1016/j.tifs.2020.03.018]

[12]   Hardman R, Fazli F. Methods of screening the genus Trigonella for steroidal sapogenins in genus Trigonella. Planta medi 1972; 21(02): 131-8.

[13]   Akhtar N, Waqas M, Ahmed M, *et al.* Effect of cream formulation of fenugreek seed extract on some mechanical parameters of human skin. Trop J Pharm Res 2010; 9(4): 329-37.
[http://dx.doi.org/10.4314/tjpr.v9i4.58922]

[14]   Acharya S, Thomas J, Basu S. Fenugreek, an alternative crop for semiarid regions of North America. Crop Sci 2008; 48(3): 841-53.
[http://dx.doi.org/10.2135/cropsci2007.09.0519]

[15]   Basu A, Basu SK, Kumar A, *et al.* Fenugreek (*Trigonella foenum-graecum* L.), a potential new crop for Latin America. Am J Social Issues and Humanities 2014; 4(3): 147-62.

[16]   Petropoulos G. Fenugreek-The genus Trigonella. London, New York: Taylor and Francis 2002.
[http://dx.doi.org/10.4324/9780203217474]

[17]   Basu T, Srichamroen A. Health Benefits of Fenugreek (*Trigonella-foenum-graecum Leguminosse*) Watson RR, Preedy VR. Bioactive foods in promoting health. Amsterdam: Academic Press 2010.

[18]   Bouhenni H, Doukani K, Şekeroğlu N, Gezici S, Tabak S. Comparative study on chemical composition and antibacterial activity of fenugreek (*Trigonella Foenum graecum* L.) and cumin (*Cuminum cyminum* L.) seeds. Ukr Food J 2019; 8(4): 755-67.
[http://dx.doi.org/10.24263/2304-974X-2019-8-4-7]

[19]   Dwivedi G, Singh S, Giri D. Effect of varieties and processing on nutritional composition of fenugreek seeds. J Pharm Innov 2019; 8(12): 68-72.

[20]   El Bairi K, Ouzir M, Agnieszka N, Khalki L. Anticancer potential of *Trigonella foenum graecum*: Cellular and molecular targets. Biomed Pharmacother 2017; 90: 479-91.
[http://dx.doi.org/10.1016/j.biopha.2017.03.071] [PMID: 28391170]

[21]   Liu F, Chang W, Chen M, Xu F, Ma J, Zhong F. Film-forming properties of guar gum, tara gum and locust bean gum. Food Hydrocoll 2020.98105007.
[http://dx.doi.org/10.1016/j.foodhyd.2019.03.028]

[22]   Stephen AM, Phillips GO. Food polysaccharides and their applications. CRC press 2016; p. 750.
[http://dx.doi.org/10.1201/9781420015164]

[23]   Qin X, Li R, Zhu S, *et al.* A comparative study of sulfated tara gum: RSM optimization and structural characterization. Int J Biol Macromol 2020; 150: 189-99.
[http://dx.doi.org/10.1016/j.ijbiomac.2020.02.031] [PMID: 32050084]

[24]   Dakia PA, Blecker C, Robert C, Wathelet B, Paquot M. Composition and physicochemical properties of locust bean gum extracted from whole seeds by acid or water dehulling pre-treatment. Food Hydrocoll 2008; 22(5): 807-18.
[http://dx.doi.org/10.1016/j.foodhyd.2007.03.007]

[25]   Gidley MJ, Reid JG. Chapter-6. Galactomannans and other cell wall storage polysaccharides in seeds. Food polysaccharides and their applications 2006; 181-216.

[26]   Salarbashi D, Bazeli J, Fahmideh-Rad E. Fenugreek seed gum: Biological properties, chemical modifications, and structural analysis- A review. Int J Biol Macromol 2019; 138: 386-93.
[http://dx.doi.org/10.1016/j.ijbiomac.2019.07.006] [PMID: 31276725]

[27]   Anwar S, Desai S, Mandlik R. Exploring antidiabetic mechanisms of action of galactomannan: A carbohydrate isolated from fenugreek seeds. J Complement Integr Med 2009; 6(1): 1-6.

[http://dx.doi.org/10.2202/1553-3840.1218]

[28] Sundaram G, Theagarajan R, Gopalakrishnan K, Babu GR, Murthy GD. Effect of fenugreek consumption with metformin treatment in improving plaque index in diabetic patients. J Nat Sci Biol Med 2020; 11(1): 55-60.
[http://dx.doi.org/10.4103/jnsbm.JNSBM_96_19]

[29] Kamble H, Kandhare AD, Bodhankar S, Mohan V, Thakurdesai P. Effect of low molecular weight galactomannans from fenugreek seeds on animal models of diabetes mellitus. Biomed Aging Pathol 2013; 3(3): 145-51.
[http://dx.doi.org/10.1016/j.biomag.2013.06.002]

[30] Shashikumar J, Champawat P, Mudgal V, Jain S. Role of fenugreek (*Trigonella foenum graecum*) on in management of diabetes disease. J Pharmacogn Phytochem 2019; 8(4): 184-7.

[31] Singh B, Singh JP, Singh N, Kaur A. Saponins in pulses and their health promoting activities: A review. Food Chem 2017; 233: 540-9.
[http://dx.doi.org/10.1016/j.foodchem.2017.04.161] [PMID: 28530610]

[32] Oleszek M, Oleszek W. Saponins in Food. Handbook of Dietary Phytochemicals. 2020; pp. 1-40.
[http://dx.doi.org/10.1007/978-981-13-1745-3_34-1]

[33] Waller GR, Yamasaki K. Chapter-1. Saponins used in traditional and modern medicine. New York: Springer Science & Business Media 2013.

[34] Marrelli M, Conforti F, Araniti F, Statti GA. Effects of saponins on lipid metabolism: A review of potential health benefits in the treatment of obesity. Molecules 2016; 21(10): 1404-24.
[http://dx.doi.org/10.3390/molecules21101404] [PMID: 27775618]

[35] Reddy R, Gowda A, Srinivasan K. Antilithogenic and hypocholesterolemic effect of dietary fenugreek seeds (*Trigonella foenum-graecum*) in experimental mice. Medicinal Plants-Int J Phytomed Related Ind 2019; 11(2): 145-54.
[http://dx.doi.org/10.5958/0975-6892.2019.00018.2]

[36] Belguith-Hadriche O, Bouaziz M, Jamoussi K, El Feki A, Sayadi S, Makni-Ayedi F. Lipid-lowering and antioxidant effects of an ethyl acetate extract of fenugreek seeds in high-cholesterol-fed rats. J Agric Food Chem 2010; 58(4): 2116-22.
[http://dx.doi.org/10.1021/jf903186w] [PMID: 20108903]

[37] Avalos-Soriano A, De la Cruz-Cordero R, Rosado JL, Garcia-Gasca T. 4-Hydroxyisoleucine from fenugreek (*Trigonella foenum-graecum*): Effects on insulin resistance associated with obesity. Molecules 2016; 21(11): 1596-606.
[http://dx.doi.org/10.3390/molecules21111596] [PMID: 27879673]

[38] Broca C, Breil V, Cruciani-Guglielmacci C, *et al.* Insulinotropic agent ID-1101 (4-hydroxyisoleucine) activates insulin signaling in rat. Am J Physiol Endocrinol Metab 2004; 287(3): E463-71.
[http://dx.doi.org/10.1152/ajpendo.00163.2003] [PMID: 15082420]

[39] Ogawa J, Kodera T, Smirnov SV, *et al.* A novel L-isoleucine metabolism in Bacillus thuringiensis generating (2S,3R,4S)-4-hydroxyisoleucine, a potential insulinotropic and anti-obesity amino acid. Appl Microbiol Biotechnol 2011; 89(6): 1929-38.
[http://dx.doi.org/10.1007/s00253-010-2983-7] [PMID: 21069315]

[40] Shi F, Zhang S, Li Y, Lu Z. Enhancement of substrate supply and ido expression to improve 4-hydroxyisoleucine production in recombinant *Corynebacterium glutamicum* ssp. *lactofermentum.* Appl Microbiol Biotechnol 2019; 103(10): 4113-24.
[http://dx.doi.org/10.1007/s00253-019-09791-2] [PMID: 30953121]

[41] Garg RC. Fenugreek: multiple health benefits.Nutraceuticals. Elsevier 2016; pp. 599-617.

[42] Nugrahini AD, Ishida M, Nakagawa T, Nishi K, Sugahara T. Trigonelline: An alkaloid with anti-degranulation properties. Mol Immunol 2020; 118: 201-9.
[http://dx.doi.org/10.1016/j.molimm.2019.12.020] [PMID: 31896496]

[43]   Costa MC, Lima TFO, Arcaro CA, *et al.* Trigonelline and curcumin alone, but not in combination, counteract oxidative stress and inflammation and increase glycation product detoxification in the liver and kidney of mice with high-fat diet-induced obesity. J Nutr Biochem 2020; 76108303.
[http://dx.doi.org/10.1016/j.jnutbio.2019.108303] [PMID: 76108303.]

[44]   Haouala R, Hawala S, El-Ayeb A, Khanfir R, Boughanmi N. Aqueous and organic extracts of *Trigonella foenum-graecum* L. inhibit the mycelia growth of fungi. J Environ Sci (China) 2008; 20(12): 1453-7.
[http://dx.doi.org/10.1016/S1001-0742(08)62548-6] [PMID: 19209631]

[45]   Oddepally R, Guruprasad L. Isolation, purification, and characterization of a stable defensin-like antifungal peptide from *Trigonella foenum-graecum* (fenugreek) seeds. Biochemistry (Mosc) 2015; 80(3): 332-42.
[http://dx.doi.org/10.1134/S0006297915030086] [PMID: 25761687]

[46]   Sulieman AME, Ahmed HE, Abdelrahim AM. The chemical composition of fenugreek (*Trigonella foenum graceu*m L) and the antimicrobial properties of its seed oil. Gezira J Eng Appl Sci 2008; 3(2): 52-71.

[47]   Das S, Anjeza C, Mandal S. Synergistic or additive antimicrobial activities of Indian spice and herbal extracts against pathogenic, probiotic and food-spoiler micro-organisms. Int Food Res J 2012; 19(3): 1185-91.

[48]   Wagh P, Rai M, Deshmukh S, Durate MCT. Bio-activity of oils of *Trigonella foenum-graecum* and Pongamia pinnata. Afr J Biotechnol 2007; 6(13): 1592-6.

[49]   Prusky D, McEvoy JL, Saftner R, Conway WS, Jones R. Relationship between host acidification and virulence of *Penicillium* spp. on apple and citrus fruit. Phytopathology 2004; 94(1): 44-51.
[http://dx.doi.org/10.1094/PHYTO.2004.94.1.44] [PMID: 18943818]

[50]   Saini P, Dubey N, Singh P, Singh A. Effect of processing methods on proximate composition and antioxidant activity of fenugreek (*Trigonella foenum-graecum*) seeds. Int J Agric Food Sci 2016; 6: 82-7.

[51]   Walli RR, Al-Musrati RA, Eshtewi HM, Sherif FM. Screening of antimicrobial activity of fenugreek seeds. Pharm Pharmacol Int J 2015; 2(4): 1-4.

[52]   Mehani M, Segni L. Antimicrobial effect of essential oil of plant *Trigonella foenum-graecum* on some bacteria pathogens. World Academy of Science, Engineering and Technology, International Journal of Medical, Health, Biomedical Bioengineering and Pharmaceutical Engineering 2012; 6(9): 430-42.

[53]   Dash B, Sultana S, Sultana N. Antibacterial activities of methanol and acetone extracts of fenugreek (*Trigonella foenum*) and coriander (*Coriandrum sativum*). Life Sci Med Res 2011; 27: 1-8.

[54]   Dubey R, Dubey K, Janapati YK, Sridhar C, Jayaveera K. Comparative anti microbial studies of aqueous, methanolic and saponins extract of seeds of *Trigonella foenum-graecum* on human vaginal pathogens causing UTI infection. Pharma Chem 2010; 2(5): 84-8.

[55]   Ritu K, Atanu C, Pal SB, Ashutosh G, Kalyan S. Antimicrobial activity of ethanolic extract of *Trigonella foenum-graecum* Linn. Int Res J Pharm 2010; 1(1): 181-3.

[56]   Deshmukh AR, Gupta A, Kim BS. Ultrasound assisted green synthesis of silver and iron oxide nanoparticles using fenugreek seed extract and their enhanced antibacterial and antioxidant activities. BioMed Res Int 2019; 20191714358.
[http://dx.doi.org/10.1155/2019/1714358] [PMID: 31080808]

[57]   Yasmeen R, Shashikumar J. Fenugreek (*Trigonella foenum-graecum*) and its Antimicrobial Activity-A Review. Int J Curr Microbiol Appl Sci 2019; 8(6): 710-24.
[http://dx.doi.org/10.20546/ijcmas.2019.806.083]

[58]   Kanan G, Al-Najar R. *In vitro* and *in vivo* activity of selected plant crude extracts and fractions against *Penicillium italicum.* J Plant Prot Res 2009; 49(4): 341-52.

[http://dx.doi.org/10.2478/v10045-009-0054-9]

[59]   Nandagopal S, Dhanalakshmi D, Kumar AG, Sujitha D. Phytochemical and antibacterial studies of fenugreek *Trigonella foenum-graecum* L.-A multipurpose medicinal plant. J Pharm Res 2012; 5(1): 413-5.

[60]   Wani SA, Kumar P. Fenugreek: A review on its nutraceutical properties and utilization in various food products. J Saudi Soc Agric Sci 2018; 17(2): 97-106.
[http://dx.doi.org/10.1016/j.jssas.2016.01.007]

[61]   Tharaheswari M, Jayachandra Reddy N, Kumar R, Varshney KC, Kannan M, Sudha Rani S. Trigonelline and diosgenin attenuate ER stress, oxidative stress-mediated damage in pancreas and enhance adipose tissue PPARγ activity in type 2 diabetic rats. Mol Cell Biochem 2014; 396(1-2): 161-74.
[http://dx.doi.org/10.1007/s11010-014-2152-x] [PMID: 25070833]

[62]   Jung D-H, Park H-J, Byun H-E, *et al.* Diosgenin inhibits macrophage-derived inflammatory mediators through downregulation of CK2, JNK, NF-kappaB and AP-1 activation. Int Immunopharmacol 2010; 10(9): 1047-54.
[http://dx.doi.org/10.1016/j.intimp.2010.06.004] [PMID: 20601188]

[63]   Maurya CK, Singh R, Jaiswal N, Venkateswarlu K, Narender T, Tamrakar AK. 4-Hydroxyisoleucine ameliorates fatty acid-induced insulin resistance and inflammatory response in skeletal muscle cells. Mol Cell Endocrinol 2014; 395(1-2): 51-60.
[http://dx.doi.org/10.1016/j.mce.2014.07.018] [PMID: 25109277]

[64]   Venkatesan N, Devaraj SN, Devaraj H. A fibre cocktail of fenugreek, guar gum and wheat bran reduces oxidative modification of LDL induced by an atherogenic diet in rats. Mol Cell Biochem 2007; 294(1-2): 145-53.
[http://dx.doi.org/10.1007/s11010-006-9254-z] [PMID: 16855793]

[65]   Belguith-Hadriche O, Bouaziz M, Jamoussi K, Simmonds MS, El Feki A, Makni-Ayedi F. Comparative study on hypocholesterolemic and antioxidant activities of various extracts of fenugreek seeds. Food Chem 2013; 138(2-3): 1448-53.
[http://dx.doi.org/10.1016/j.foodchem.2012.11.003] [PMID: 23411266]

[66]   Kaviarasan S, Naik GH, Gangabhagirathi R, Anuradha CV, Priyadarsini KI. *In vitro* studies on antiradical and antioxidant activities of fenugreek (*Trigonella foenum graecum*) seeds. Food Chem 2007; 103(1): 31-7.
[http://dx.doi.org/10.1016/j.foodchem.2006.05.064]

[67]   Tavakoly R, Maracy MR, Karimifar M, Entezari MH. Does fenugreek (*Trigonella foenum-graecum*) seed improve inflammation, and oxidative stress in patients with type 2 diabetes mellitus? A parallel group randomized clinical trial. Eur J Integr Med 2018; 18: 13-7.
[http://dx.doi.org/10.1016/j.eujim.2018.01.005]

[68]   Mukthamba P, Srinivasan K. Dietary fenugreek (*Trigonella foenum-graecum*) seeds and garlic (*Allium sativum*) alleviates oxidative stress in experimental myocardial infarction. Food Sci Hum Wellness 2017; 6(2): 77-87.
[http://dx.doi.org/10.1016/j.fshw.2017.04.001]

[69]   Baba WN, Tabasum Q, Muzzaffar S, Masoodi FA, Wani I, Ganie SA, *et al.* Some nutraceutical properties of fenugreek seeds and shoots (*Trigonella foenum-graecum* L.) from the high Himalayan region. Food Biosci 2018; 23: 31-7.
[http://dx.doi.org/10.1016/j.fbio.2018.02.009]

[70]   Akbari S, Abdurahman NH, Yunus RM, Alara OR, Abayomi OO. Extraction, characterization and antioxidant activity of fenugreek (*Trigonella-foenum graecum*) seed oil. Material Sci Energy Technol 2019; 2(2): 349-55.
[http://dx.doi.org/10.1016/j.mset.2018.12.001]

[71]   Kaveh S, Sadeghi M, Ghorbani M, Jafari M. Sarabandi k. Optimization of factors affecting the

antioxidant activity of fenugreek seed's protein hydrolysate by response surface methodology. Iran J Nutr Sci Food Technol 2019; 14(1): 77-87.

[72] Subramanian SP, Prasath GS. Antidiabetic and antidyslipidemic nature of trigonelline, a major alkaloid of fenugreek seeds studied in high-fat-fed and low-dose streptozotocin-induced experimental diabetic rats. Biomed Preven Nutri 2014; 4(4): 475-80.
[http://dx.doi.org/10.1016/j.bionut.2014.07.001]

[73] Robert SD, Ismail AA, Rosli WIW. Reduction of postprandial blood glucose in healthy subjects by buns and flatbreads incorporated with fenugreek seed powder. Eur J Nutr 2016; 55(7): 2275-80.
[http://dx.doi.org/10.1007/s00394-015-1037-4] [PMID: 26358163]

[74] Jin Y, Shi Y, Zou Y, Miao C, Sun B, Li C. Fenugreek prevents the development of STZ-induced diabetic nephropathy in a rat model of diabetes. Evid Based Complement Alternat Med 2014; 2014259368.
[http://dx.doi.org/10.1155/2014/259368] [PMID: 2014259368.]

[75] Singh AB, Tamarkar AK, Narender T, Srivastava AK. Antihyperglycaemic effect of an unusual amino acid (4-hydroxyisoleucine) in C57BL/KsJ-db/db mice. Nat Prod Res 2010; 24(3): 258-65.
[http://dx.doi.org/10.1080/14786410902836693] [PMID: 20140804]

[76] Hadi A, Arab A, Hajianfar H, *et al.* The effect of fenugreek seed supplementation on serum irisin levels, blood pressure, and liver and kidney function in patients with type 2 diabetes mellitus: A parallel randomized clinical trial. Complement Ther Med 2020; 49102315.
[http://dx.doi.org/10.1016/j.ctim.2020.102315] [PMID: 32147060]

[77] Geberemeskel GA, Debebe YG, Nguse NA. Antidiabetic effect of fenugreek seed powder solution (*Trigonella foenum-graecum* L.) on hyperlipidemia in diabetic patients. J Diabetes Res 2019.20198507453.
[http://dx.doi.org/10.1155/2019/8507453] [PMID: 31583253]

[78] Dalvi SM, Patwardhan MS, Yeram N, Patil VW, Patwardhan SY. Evaluation of biochemical markers in type 2 diabetes mellitus with adjunct therapy of fenugreek seed aqueous extract. J Med Plants Stud 2019; 7(1): 109-13.

[79] Sindhu G, Ratheesh M, Shyni GL, Nambisan B, Helen A. Anti-inflammatory and antioxidative effects of mucilage of *Trigonella foenum graecum* (Fenugreek) on adjuvant induced arthritic rats. Int Immunopharmacol 2012; 12(1): 205-11.
[http://dx.doi.org/10.1016/j.intimp.2011.11.012] [PMID: 22155102]

[80] Khalili M, Alavi M, Esmaeil-Jamaat E, Baluchnejadmojarad T, Roghani M. Trigonelline mitigates lipopolysaccharide-induced learning and memory impairment in the rat due to its anti-oxidative and anti-inflammatory effect. Int Immunopharmacol 2018; 61: 355-62.
[http://dx.doi.org/10.1016/j.intimp.2018.06.019] [PMID: 29935483]

[81] Mandegary A, Pournamdari M, Sharififar F, Pournourmohammadi S, Fardiar R, Shooli S. Alkaloid and flavonoid rich fractions of fenugreek seeds (*Trigonella foenum-graecum* L.) with antinociceptive and anti-inflammatory effects. Food Chem Toxicol 2012; 50(7): 2503-7.
[http://dx.doi.org/10.1016/j.fct.2012.04.020] [PMID: 22542922]

[82] Pundarikakshudu K, Shah DH, Panchal AH, Bhavsar GC. Anti-inflammatory activity of fenugreek (*Trigonella foenum-graecum* Linn) seed petroleum ether extract. Indian J Pharmacol 2016; 48(4): 441-4.
[http://dx.doi.org/10.4103/0253-7613.186195] [PMID: 27756958]

[83] Lee W, Lee D, Han E, Choi J. Intake of green tea products and obesity in nondiabetic overweight and obese females: A systematic review and meta-analysis. J Funct Foods 2019; 58: 330-7.
[http://dx.doi.org/10.1016/j.jff.2019.05.010]

[84] Figueiredo MS, Vettorazzi JF, Branco RCS, Carneiro EM. Chapter 11 - Nutrients and Obesity.Nutrition in the Prevention and Treatment of Abdominal Obesity (Second Edition). Academic Press 2019; pp. 113-21.

[85] Kumar P, Bhandari U, Jamadagni S. Fenugreek seed extract inhibit fat accumulation and ameliorates dyslipidemia in high fat diet-induced obese rats. BioMed Res Int 2014; 2014606021
[http://dx.doi.org/10.1155/2014/606021] [PMID: 24868532]

[86] Ilavenil S, Arasu MV, Lee J-C, *et al.* Trigonelline attenuates the adipocyte differentiation and lipid accumulation in 3T3-L1 cells. Phytomedicine 2014; 21(5): 758-65.
[http://dx.doi.org/10.1016/j.phymed.2013.11.007] [PMID: 24369814]

[87] Vijayakumar MV, Pandey V, Mishra GC, Bhat MK. Hypolipidemic effect of fenugreek seeds is mediated through inhibition of fat accumulation and upregulation of LDL receptor. Obesity (Silver Spring) 2010; 18(4): 667-74.
[http://dx.doi.org/10.1038/oby.2009.337] [PMID: 19851306]

[88] Uemura T, Goto T, Kang MS, *et al.* Diosgenin, the main aglycon of fenugreek, inhibits LXRα activity in HepG2 cells and decreases plasma and hepatic triglycerides in obese diabetic mice. J Nutr 2011; 141(1): 17-23.
[http://dx.doi.org/10.3945/jn.110.125591] [PMID: 21106928]

[89] Siegel RL, Miller KD, Jemal A. Cancer statistics CA: A Cancer J Clini 2019; 69(1): 7-34.

[90] Abas A-SM, Naguib DM. Effect of germination on anticancer activity of *Trigonella foenum* seeds extract. Biocatal Agric Biotechnol 2019; 18101067.
[http://dx.doi.org/10.1016/j.bcab.2019.101067]

[91] Shabbeer S, Sobolewski M, Anchoori RK, *et al.* Fenugreek: a naturally occurring edible spice as an anticancer agent. Cancer Biol Ther 2009; 8(3): 272-8.
[http://dx.doi.org/10.4161/cbt.8.3.7443] [PMID: 19197146]

[92] Stewart J, Manmathan G, Wilkinson P. Primary prevention of cardiovascular disease: A review of contemporary guidance and literature. JRSM Cardiovasc Dis 2017; 662048004016687211.
[http://dx.doi.org/10.1177/2048004016687211] [PMID: 28286646]

[93] 2016.
http://www.euro.who.int/en/health-topics/noncommunicable-diseases/cardiovascular-diseases/data-and-statistics

[94] Sharma MS, Choudhary PR. Effect of Fenugreek Seeds Powder (*Trigonella foenum-graecum* L.) on Experimental Induced Hyperlipidemia in Rabbits. J Diet Suppl 2017; 14(1): 1-8.
[http://dx.doi.org/10.3109/19390211.2016.1168905] [PMID: 27070043]

[95] Ramulu P, Giridharan NV, Udayasekhararao P. Hypolipidemic effect of soluble dietary fiber (galactomannan) isolated from fenugreek seeds in WNIN (GR-Ob) obese rats. J Med Plants Res 2011; 5(19): 4804-13.

[96] Rocha EM, De Miranda B, Sanders LH. Alpha-synuclein: Pathology, mitochondrial dysfunction and neuroinflammation in Parkinson's disease. Neurobiol Dis 2018; 109(Pt B): 249-57.
[http://dx.doi.org/10.1016/j.nbd.2017.04.004] [PMID: 28400134]

[97] Gaur V, Bodhankar SL, Mohan V, Thakurdesai P. Antidepressant-like effect of 4-hydroxyisoleucine from *Trigonella foenum graecum* L. seeds in mice. Biomed Aging Pathol 2012; 2(3): 121-5.
[http://dx.doi.org/10.1016/j.biomag.2012.07.002]

[98] Makowska J, Szczesny D, Lichucka A, Giełdoń A, Chmurzyński L, Kaliszan R. Preliminary studies on trigonelline as potential anti-Alzheimer disease agent: determination by hydrophilic interaction liquid chromatography and modeling of interactions with beta-amyloid. J Chromatogr B Analyt Technol Biomed Life Sci 2014; 968: 101-4.
[http://dx.doi.org/10.1016/j.jchromb.2013.12.001] [PMID: 24374010]

[99] Khalil WK, Roshdy HM, Kassem SM. The potential therapeutic role of Fenugreek saponin against Alzheimer's disease: Evaluation of apoptotic and acetylcholinesterase inhibitory activities. J Appl Pharm 2016; 6(09): 166-73.
[http://dx.doi.org/10.7324/JAPS.2016.60925]

[100] Anjaneyulu K, Rai KS, Rajesh T, Nagamma T, Bhat KM. Therapeutic Efficacy of Fenugreek Extract or/and Choline with Docosahexaenoic Acid in Attenuating Learning and Memory Deficits in Ovariectomized Rats. Journal of Krishna Institute of Medical Sciences University 2018; 7(2): 10-20.

[101] Araya EM, Adamu BA, Periasamy G, Sintayehu B, Gebrelibanos Hiben M. *in vivo* hepatoprotective and *In vitro* radical scavenging activities of *Cucumis ficifolius* A. rich root extract. J Ethnopharmacol 2019; 242112031.
[http://dx.doi.org/10.1016/j.jep.2019.112031] [PMID: 31220599]

[102] Feki A, Jaballi I, Cherif B, *et al.* Therapeutic potential of polysaccharide extracted from fenugreek seeds against thiamethoxam-induced hepatotoxicity and genotoxicity in Wistar adult rats. Toxicol Mech Methods 2019; 29(5): 355-67.
[http://dx.doi.org/10.1080/15376516.2018.1564949] [PMID: 30621503]

[103] Kaviarasan S, Anuradha CV. Fenugreek (*Trigonella foenum graecum*) seed polyphenols protect liver from alcohol toxicity: a role on hepatic detoxification system and apoptosis. Pharmazie 2007; 62(4): 299-304.
[PMID: 17484288]

[104] Belaïd-Nouira Y, Bakhta H, Haouas Z, *et al.* Fenugreek seeds, a hepatoprotector forage crop against chronic AlCl3 toxicity. BMC Vet Res 2013; 9(1): 22.
[http://dx.doi.org/10.1186/1746-6148-9-22] [PMID: 23363543]

[105] Arlt A, Sebens S, Krebs S, *et al.* Inhibition of the Nrf2 transcription factor by the alkaloid trigonelline renders pancreatic cancer cells more susceptible to apoptosis through decreased proteasomal gene expression and proteasome activity. Oncogene 2013; 32(40): 4825-35.
[http://dx.doi.org/10.1038/onc.2012.493] [PMID: 23108405]

[106] Mohammad-Sadeghipour M, Mahmoodi M, Falahati-pour SK, Khoshdel A, Fahmidehkar MA, Mirzaei MR, *et al. Trigonella foenum-graecum* seed extract modulates expression of lipid metabolism-related genes in HepG2 cells. Asian Pac J Trop Biomed 2019; 9(6): 240-8.
[http://dx.doi.org/10.4103/2221-1691.260396]

[107] Snehlata HS, Payal DR. Fenugreek (*Trigonella foenum-graecum* L.): an overview. Int J Curr Pharm Rev Res 2012; 2(4): 169-87.

[108] Işıklı ND, Karababa E. Rheological characterization of fenugreek paste (çemen). J Food Eng 2005; 69(2): 185-90.
[http://dx.doi.org/10.1016/j.jfoodeng.2004.08.013]

[109] Hegazy A, Ibrahium M. Evaluation of the nutritional protein quality of wheat biscuit supplemented by fenugreek seed flour. World J Dairy Food Sci 2009; 4(2): 129-35.

[110] Hussein A, Amal S, Amany M, Abeer A, Gamal H. Physiochemical, sensory and nutritional properties of corn-fenugreek flour composite biscuits. Aust J Basic Appl Sci 2011; 5(4): 84-95.

[111] Wani S, Kumar P. Fenugreek enriched extruded product: optimization of ingredients using response surface methodology. Int Food Res J 2016; 23(1): 18-25.

[112] Bakr A. Production of iron□fortified bread employing some selected natural iron sources. Food/Nahrung 1997; 41(5): 293-8.
[http://dx.doi.org/10.1002/food.19970410509]

[113] Galal OM. The nutrition transition in Egypt: obesity, undernutrition and the food consumption context. Public Health Nutr 2002; 5(1A): 141-8.
[http://dx.doi.org/10.1079/PHN2001286] [PMID: 12027277]

[114] Sharma H, Chauhan G. Effects of stabilized rice bran: fenugreek blends on the quality of breads and cookies. J Food Sci Technol 2002; 39(3): 225-33.

[115] Yamani N. Formulation and evaluation of polyherbal hair oil. J Pharm Phytochem 2018; 7(3): 3254-6.

[116] Noudeh GD, Sharififar F, Khazaeli P, Mohajeri E, Jahanbakhsh J. Formulation of herbal conditioner

shampoo by using extract of fenugreek seeds and evaluation of its physicochemical parameters. Afr J Pharm Pharmacol 2011; 5(22): 2420-7.

[117] Mamoun T, Mukhtar MA, Tabidi MH. Effect of fenugreek seed powder on the performance, carcass characteristics and some blood serum attributes. Adv Res Agri Vet Sci 2014; 1(1): 6-11.

[118] Hegazy A. Influence of using fenugreek seed flour as antioxidant and antimicrobial agent in the manufacturing of beef burger with emphasis on frozen storage stability. World J Agric Sci 2011; 7(4): 391-9.

[119] Mikkonen KS, Tenkanen M, Cooke P, *et al.* Mannans as stabilizers of oil-in-water beverage emulsions. Lebensm Wiss Technol 2009; 42(4): 849-55.
[http://dx.doi.org/10.1016/j.lwt.2008.11.010]

[120] Aruna R, Manjula B, Penchalaraju Mand Chandrika C. Effect of fenugreek seed mucilage on physico-chemical properties of Mosambi fruit juice. J Pharmacognosy Phytochem 2018; 7(1): 1887-90.

[121] Kandhare AD, Thakurdesai PA, Wangikar P, Bodhankar SL. A systematic literature review of fenugreek seed toxicity by using ToxRTool: evidence from preclinical and clinical studies. Heliyon 2019; 5(4)e01536.
[http://dx.doi.org/10.1016/j.heliyon.2019.e01536] [PMID: 31049444]

[122] Al-Yahya AA. Reproductive, cytological and biochemical toxicity of fenugreek in male Swiss albino mice. Afr J Pharm Pharmacol 2013; 7(29): 2072-80.
[http://dx.doi.org/10.5897/AJPP2013.3449]

[123] Ibrahim M, El-Tawill G. Possible outcome of fenugreek seeds powder administration on the fertility of female and male albino rat. J Rad Res Appl Sci 2010; 3(2): 357-72.

[124] Aswar U, Bodhankar SL, Mohan V, Thakurdesai PA. Effect of furostanol glycosides from *Trigonella foenum-graecum* on the reproductive system of male albino rats. Phytother Res 2010; 24(10): 1482-8.
[http://dx.doi.org/10.1002/ptr.3129] [PMID: 20878698]

[125] Swaroop A, Bagchi M, Kumar P, *et al.* Safety, efficacy and toxicological evaluation of a novel, patented anti-diabetic extract of *Trigonella foenum-graecum* seed extract (Fenfuro). Toxicol Mech Methods 2014; 24(7): 495-503.
[http://dx.doi.org/10.3109/15376516.2014.943443] [PMID: 25045923]

[126] Khalki L, M'hamed SB, Bennis M, Chait A, Sokar Z. Evaluation of the developmental toxicity of the aqueous extract from *Trigonella foenum-graecum* (L.) in mice. J Ethnopharmacol 2010; 131(2): 321-5.
[http://dx.doi.org/10.1016/j.jep.2010.06.033] [PMID: 20600755]

CHAPTER 5

Biological Activities of *Foeniculum vulgare* Mill.

Anitha Rajasekaran[*]

Department of Botany, Bharathi Women's College, Prakasam Salai, Broadway, Chennai-600108, India

Abstract: In recent years, traditional systems of medicine are widely practiced throughout the world to treat various ailments that have originated due to the rise in population, increase in the cost of the drug, side effects of synthetic drugs and emergence of drug resistance in microbes. Asian food contains various culinary herbs that are used extensively in the traditional systems of medicine. One such important oldest culinary herb is *Foeniculum vulgare* Mill. It is an annual herb (Apiaceae), cultivated as arid and semiarid crop in the tropics and temperate regions of the world. Today, it finds its application in the healthcare industry, pharmaceutics, food, and cosmetics. Major components of *F. vulgare* essential oil are trans-anethole, estragole (methyl chavicol), fenchone and phellandrene. They also contain fatty acids, phenylpropanoids, terpene, coumarins, tannins, flavonoids, cardiac glycosides, and saponins. It is reported to possess antimicrobial, antiviral, antimycobacterial, antiprotozoal,anti-infantile, anti-inflammatory, antipyretic, antimutagenic, antihirsutim, antinociceptive, antispasmodic chemo modulatory, antitumor, antithrombotic, apoptotic hepatoprotective, hypolipidemic, hypoglycemic, memory enhancing and oestrogenic properties. It also has antioxidant, cytotoxic, bronchodilatory, diuretic, galactagogue, emmenagogue, hypotensive and gastroprotective activities. Due to its antioxidant properties, it has lesser side effects and also reduce toxicity. Hence, it can be used effectively in combating various diseases. This chapter presents a comprehensive summary of the various biological activities of *F. vulgare*.

Keywords: Anethole, Biological activities, Culinary herb, Essential oils, *Foeniculum vulgare*, Limonene, Pharmacological activities.

INTRODUCTION

Since prehistoric time, man has witnessed the use of herbs to treat various ailments. During the last two decades, the use of herbs either as complementary or alternative medicine has increased. According to WHO, about 80% of the world's population depends on traditional systems of medicine. Natural remedies and herbal medicine are cost-effective with lesser adverse effects. Moreover, natural

[*] **Corresponding Author Anitha Rajasekaran:** Department of Botany, Bharathi Women's College, Prakasam Salai, Broadway, Chennai-600108, India; Tel: 91-044-26268358; E-mail anitha.rajasekaran023@gmail.com

Atta-ur-Rahman, M. Iqbal Choudhary & Sammer Yousuf

compounds induce a biological balance and avoid drug retention [1]. Medicinal plants act as repositories of bioactive compounds. The bioactive compounds in plants act synergistically to bring about a specific effect. Over 4,2,000 flowering plants have been discovered around the world. More than 5,000 plants are reported to have medicinal uses. Among these plants, *Foeniculum vulgare* Mill contains a large number of phytochemicals with different biological activities [2].

Fennel is an important crop with enormous usage in medicine and industrial fields. It is used in pharmaceuticals, food, flavoring agent in products such as liqueurs, bread, cheese, cosmetics, and health care industries. It is the oldest spice cultivated throughout the world as a medicinal herb, essential oil plant or as a vegetable. Approximately 20% of its production is exported to the Middle East, Europe and the USA [3].

Apart from the diverse phytochemicals that are responsible for various biological activities, other constituents of fennel are mineral and trace elements such as, nickel, lead, strontium, zinc, magnesium, manganese, aluminum, barium, calcium, chromium, cadmium, cobalt, copper and iron [4]; water-soluble vitamins like ascorbic acid, riboflavin, thiamine, niacin and pyridoxine; fat-soluble vitamins A, E, and K and essential amino acids leucine, isoleucine, phenylalanine, and tryptophan contribute to the enormous health benefits.

Distribution

F. vulgare originates from southern Europe and Asia. It is grown in Algeria, Argentina, Afghanistan, Africa, Albania, Australia, Bosnia, Bulgaria, Brazil, Costa Rica, Chile, Croatia, Egypt, France, Guatemala, Greece, Georgia, Herzegovina, Iran, Iraq, India, Italy, Jordan, Libya, Lebanon, Montenegro, Morocco, Mexico, New Zealand, Pakistan, Portugal, Palestine, Paraguay, Syria, Spain, Salvador, Tunisia, Turkey, Ukraine, United Kingdom, United States, Venezuela, and Uruguay [4]. Many races and varieties differ in their colour, size, odour, and taste. Variety *vulgare* is grown extensively in many parts of the world. According to certain reports, two sub-species of fennel, *F. piperitum* and *F. vulgare* can be differentiated based on the taste and odour. Sub-species *piperitum* has bitter seeds, while *vulgare* has sweet seeds that are used as flavouring agents in baked food, meat, fish, ice creams and alcoholic beverages [5]. However, morphological differences between these two subspecies are not well defined. India is the largest producer of fennel in the world. It is cultivated in Gujarat, Rajasthan and Uttar Pradesh. It is also grown in small pockets in Karnataka, Maharashtra, Punjab, Bihar, Jammu and Kashmir.

Description

Foeniculum vulgare Mill. is a perennial, aromatic herb growing to a height of 2.5m.It has a characteristic hollow stem with finely dissected filiform leaves that are 40 cm in length and 0.5 mm in width. The inflorescence is a compound umbel with flowers borne terminally. The flowers are bright golden, bisexual, regular or irregular. The fruits are greenish-yellow,elongated, elliptical, slightly curved and obtuse at the end with 3-5 strong longitudinal ribs with persistent stylopodium. On the contrary, the wild fruits are short, intensely coloured and blunt at their ends [3]. It bears small seeds of 8mm in length and 3 mm in breadth with aromatic odour and sweet taste.

Traditional Uses

Fennel is used as a culinary herb over 4000 years. The ancient Egyptians used it as food and medicine. The Greek physicians, Hippocrates and Dioscorides reported fennel to be diuretic, emmenagogue and its juice strengthened the eyesight. It is known to increase milk production, menstruation and help in delivery of the foetus. In ancient times, the Saxon peopleconsidered it sacred and valued as a magical herb [3, 6, 7]. In the middle ages, it was used to protect households from evil spirits [8]. Fifth century discovered fennel to possess sedative effect and numerous therapeutic properties attributed to it in the 9th to 14th century [9]. Fennel is one of the most frequently quoted plants in the chilandar medical codex from the 12th to 15th century [10]. Over thousands of years, East Asian countries such as India and China have used fennel to treat various ailments. Chinese medicine regarded it as carminative, stimulant and used in relieving chills, abdominal distension, vomiting and diarrhoea. It is an excellent remedy for snakebite.

Ayurveda and Siddha considered it as a stimulant, carminative, aromatic, stomachic, emmenagogue and galactagogue; It was used as galactagogue, since the phytoestrogens in fennel are reported to enhance the growth of breast tissue in feeding mothers [11]. Poultice of fennel was used to relieve inflammation of breast in nursing mothers during lactation. A decoction of fennel was used to relieve flatulence, colic, diuretic, diaphoretic in children and infants. A hot infusion was used to treat amenorrhea and to clear liver and spleen obstructions. The fennel seeds are eaten raw, sometimes with sweetener to improve eyesight. The animal studies have shown potential use in the treatment of glaucoma and hypertension.

The Romans too believed that fennel seed strengthened vision. The English used to get rid of bloating stomach and facilitate digestion through it. Since the 18th century, therapeutic uses have been studied extensively [12]. Today, it is used to cure diabetes, bronchitis, chronic cough and kidney stones [13]. The diuretic properties of the plant have been well documented to treat kidney and bladder diseases; to treat nausea, vomiting and dyspepsia.

In the Arabian system of medicine, it is widely used as a diuretic, appetizer, and digestive stimulant [14]. The infused fruits were used as carminative. Roots were regarded as purgative. Crushed fruits were inhaled to relieve dizziness. Shoots of the young plant were used to cure gas and respiratory disorders. Decoction was gargled as a breath freshener or as eyewash. Hot infusion of fruits and roots were used for amenorrhea. Infusion of roots was administered for toothache and urinary disorder. Oil was used for flatulence and intestinal worms. A paste of seeds or fruits were used as a cooling drink in case of fever. Seeds were also used as a stimulant to enhance libido in men and for the treatment of venereal diseases [15].

Europe and Mediterranean countries used fennel as an anti-inflammatory, analgesic, antispasmodic, diuretic, galactagogue, antioxidant and as an eye lotion. The fennel powder is used as a poultice on snake bitten parts of the body and infusions used for babies to prevent flatulence and colic spasm. A subspecies of fennel, *F. vulgare* subsp. *piperitum*, is used for mouth ulcers in the Basilicata region of southern Italy in Portugal. It is used in the treatment of diabetes, bronchitis, chronic coughs and kidney stones [16, 14].

In Mexican traditional medicine, a decoction is used as a galactagogue, to treat tuberculosis and other respiratory diseases [17, 18]. In Palestine, it is a popular digestive stimulant. Fennel leaf infusion is also used to treat infant's stomachache. Guyana and Surinam adults used seeds to dispel gases. Boiled or roasted roots are effective for the treatment of gonorrhea in East Africa [19, 20]. Barks of tree used for blood-related diseases [21]. Roots were used for urinary tract infection, renal calculi and glycosuria [22].

Culinary Uses

The foliage, bulb and seeds of the plant are widely used in many cuisines of the world. It is used to flavor baked food products, herbal mixtures, alcoholic beverages and ice cream [23]. Green seeds are best used in cooking. The bulbs are generally stewed, sautéed, grilled or eaten raw. The bulbs and fronds are important ingredients in the Mediterranean cuisine, where they are eaten raw or cooked. Fennel seeds are used in Indian and Middle East cooking as well.

Phytochemical Composition of Fennel

The phytochemical components are responsible for biological activity (Table **1**). Although the entire plant is useful, seeds are used extensively [24]. The seed contains water, carbohydrates, protein, fat, minerals and fibers. Vitamins and minerals such as thiamine, riboflavin, niacin, vitamin C, calcium, potassium, sodium, iron, and phosphorus are present in the leaves [25]. Oil of fruits contains 22% oleic acid, 4% palmitic acid, 14% linoleic acid and 6% petrocylic acid. The essential oil varies according to the environment and growth of the plant [26]. It contains more than 30 types of terpene compounds. Among the terpenes, 50 to 80% trans-anethole, 8% fenchone and limonene 5% were evident in the essential oil [27]. Phenolic compounds such as phenolic acids, flavonoids, coumarin, hydroxycinnamic acids, and tannin are also present [28, 29]. Phenolic acids include 3-O-Caffeoylquinicacid, 4-O-caffeoylquinic acid, 5-O-caffeoylquinic acid, 1, 3-O-di-caffeoylquinic acid, 1,4-O-di-caffeoylquinic acid, and 1, 5-O--i-caffeoylquinic acid. Its flavonoid constituents are quercetin-3-rutinoside and rosmarinic acid [30]. Aqueous extract of fennel fruit contained quercetin-3-O-glucuronide, quercetin-3-O-galactoside, kaempferol-3-O-glucoside, kaempferol-3-O-glucuronide, kaempferol-3-O-rutinoside, isoquercetin, and isorhamnetin-3-O-glucoside [31].

Biological Activities

Antimicrobial Activity

Identifying anti-microbial agents with bioactive compounds that can significantly combat gram-positive and gram-negative infections is necessary due to the emergence of multi-drug resistance in the pathogens [32]. Shahid *et al.* [33], reported significant activity of acetone and hot aqueous extracts of the fruits on *Staphylococcus aureus,Enterococcus faecalis*, *Salmonella typhi*, *Salmonella typhimurium, Shigella flexneri, Escherichia coli*, and *Pseudomonas aeruginosa*. Weaker activity was observed with a moderate temperature of the aqueous extract; while hot extract showed negative activity. However, acetone extract showed lower Minimum Inhibitory Concentration (MIC) values than the water extract [34]. Aqueous and Ethanolic extracts of *F.vulgare* inhibited *Campylobacter jejuni* and *Helicobacter pylori* [35]. An aqueous extract of the aerial part and seeds of *F. vulgare* inhibited the growth of other bacterium such as *Agrobacterium radiobacter pv. tumefaciens, Pseudomonas fluorescens, Erwinia carotovora, Pseudomonas glycinea, Enterococcus faecalis,Escherichia coli, Staphylococcus aureus, Pseudomonas aeruginosa, Klebsiella pneumoniae, Shigella flexneri, Salmonella typhi, Salmonella typhimurium*, and *Bacillus cereus* [36, 37]. The seed extracts of diethyl ether, methanol, ethanol, and hexane were active against Gram-negative bacteria (*Escherichia coli*, and *Salmonella typhi*) and Gram-positive bacteria (*Bacillus cereus*, and *Staphylococcus aureus*).

Essential oil of fennel exhibited insignificant or moderate antibacterial activity against *E. coli*, *S. aureus*, *P. aeruginosa*, *Bacillus subtilis*, *Bacillus megaterium*, and *Bacillus cereus*, *Salmonella enteric* and *Listeria monocytogenes* [38, 39]; However, they showed synergistic activity with tetracycline or amoxicillin against *E. coli*, *B. subtilis* strains and *Sarcina lutea* [40 - 42]. Jazani *et al.* [43], reported bactericidal activity against multi-drug resistant *Acinetobacter baumannii*and agram-negative coccobacillus. Turkish essential oil was reported to be effective against *L. monocytogenes* [39], *Staphylococcus epidermidis*, *E. faecalis*, *Morganella morganii, E. coli*, *S. aureus*, *S. typhimurium*, *Salmonella enteritidis*, *Proteus mirabilis*, and *P. aeruginosa* [43]. Methanol extract had a MIC of 50 mcg/ml against 15 strains of *Helicobacter pylori* [35]. The hydro-ethanol extract was reported to be active against *Campylobacter jejuni* [44] and multidrug-resistant *Mycobacterium tuberculosis* [45]. The essential oil reduced the expression of exotoxins and enterotoxin of *S. aureus* [46]. However, *E. faecalis* and *E. coli* were found to resistant to essential oil. Phenylpropanoid derivative, Dillapional and Scopoletin (a coumarin derivative) were the antibacterial active principles identified from oil and stem respectively [47].

The aqueous and alcoholic extracts of seed were evaluated for antifungal activity against *Alternaria alternata, Mucor rouxii* and *Aspergillus flavus*. Both the extracts were completely ineffective against *Aspergillus Flavus* [48], while aqueous extract alone was very effective against *Alternaria alternata*. Aamir *et al.* [49], reported antifungal activity of acetone, ethyl acetate and chloroform extracts of unprocessed fennel on *Aspergillus, Trichoderma*, and *Metarhizium*. Both aqueous and alcoholic extracts were ineffective against *Aspergillus*, but effective against *Trichoderma* and *Metarhizium*.

The essential oil was effective on *C. albicans, A.flavus, A. niger, Fusarium-graminearum, Fusarium moniliforme* [50 - 53] dermatophyte such as *M.canis, Trichophyton rubrum, T. mentagrophytes, Microsporum gypseum*, and *T. tonsurans* [54, 55]. The activity was on par with standard antifungal agent amphotericin b and fluconazole [56]. The essential oil reduced the mycelial growth and germination of *Sclerotinia sclerotiorum*. These findings showed that essential oil of *F. vulgare* may be used as bio fungicide against phytopathogenic fungi [55]. The oils also protected stored tobacco leaves from aflatoxin contamination. Thus, it finds its application as a plant-based food preservative. The antiviral activity of essential oil was studied on the herpes simplex virus type-1 (HSV-1) and parainfluenza type-3 virus. A strong antiviral activity was evident against herpes simplex type-I only [57].

Larvicidal Activity

The methanol extract of Fennel fruit exhibited mosquito repellent activity on female *Aedes aegypti*. The repellent activity of (+)-fenchone and (E)--octadecenoic acid [58] was tested against female *Aedes aegypti* using skin and patch tests in comparison with the commercial repellent agent (N, N-diethy--toluamide (DEET) and (Z)-9-octadecenoic acid). Moderate repellent activity was evident after 30 min of treatment [59]. The larvicidal activity of the essential oils was evaluated on third instar larvae of *Aedes aegypti* for 24 h. Limonene isomers of the essential oil exhibited 99% mortality of *A. aegypti* larvae [60].

Essential oils exhibited larvicidal activity on malaria vector, *Anopheles stephensi* with LC_{50} and LC_{90} values of 20.10 and 44.51 ppm, respectively [61]. The essential oil obtained from leaves, flowers, and roots exerted larvicidal activity on fourth-instar larvae of *Culex pipiens molestus*. Terpineol and 1,8-cineole offered protection against *Culex pipiens molestus* for upto 2 hours [62]. The usage of essential oils represents a potential alternative to chemical insecticides.

Anthelmintic and Nematicidal Activity

Promising activity was evident on *D. farinae* and *D. pteronyssinus* when compared to commercial repellent such as benzyl benzoate [63]. P-anisaldehyde, thymol, estragole, (+)-fenchone and (-)-fenchone [64] were the active constituent responsible for the ascaricidal activity. Sepideh Miraj [65], investigated antischistosomal activity and cytotoxic effects against V79 cells with essential oil. Moderate *invitro* schistosomicidal activity on adult *S. mansoni* worms was evident. Remarkable inhibitory effects were observed on egg development with low toxicity [66]. Anethole and limonene in essential oils were the major constituents responsible for the inhibitory action. These constituents were active on adult *S. mansoni* worms,when compared to positive control praziquantel (PZQ) [66].

In vitro nematicidal activity of essential oils obtained from several plants were investigated. The studies revealed 80% of root-knot nematode *Meloidogyne javanica* juveniles were immobilized at a concentration of 1000 µL/liter. Hatching of the eggs was also inhibited at the same concentration [67].

Pharmacological Activities

Antioxidant Property

Oxidative stress results in the overproduction of free radicals and cause chronic degenerative diseases such as Parkinson's disease, atherosclerosis, immune dysfunction, cancer, diabetes mellitus and aging [68]. Synthetic antioxidants in food are carcinogenic and hence natural phenolic substances like phenolic acids, flavonoids and tocopherol have gained importance. These phytochemicals not only impart flavor but also increase the shelf life of food products [69]. Phytochemicals such as phenols and flavonoids are reported to possess antioxidant activity [70 - 72]. Aqueous fruit extract and four coumarins, isolated from the methanol extract, have shown excellent *In vitro* antioxidant and anti-inflammatory activities [66, 73, 74]. Musharaf Khan *et al.* [22], reported that the antioxidant property in fennel was due to polyphenols and flavonoids. Quercetin-3-O-galactoside, kaempferol-3-O-glucoside, caffeoylquinic acid, and rosmarinic acid are some of the phenolics that showed antioxidant activity.

Antioxidant activity varied in different parts of the plant. The shoots were reported to contain higher ascorbic and phenolic acid content, which explains the elevated antioxidant activity in the shoot. However, Goswami *et al.* [70], reported the presence of flavonoids in fruits. The flavonoid content varied during the stages of development. In the early stage of fruit development, flavonoid content was lower and phenolic content was higher. The infusion of fruits showed better antioxidant properties than a decoction. In addition, climatic conditions and storage period also affected the activity [75, 76]. Marino *et al.* [77], compared the antioxidant activity in fennel obtained from different Mediterranean countries. The wild fennel possessed more activity than the cultivated fennel. The volatile oil also had strong antioxidant activity and it varied with climatic regions of the world. Ahmed *et al.* [78], analyzed the essential oils of fennel obtained from Egypt and China. The Egyptian fennel contained major constituent estragole and limonene while Chinese fennel contained trans-anethole and estragole as major composition. Although both Egyptian and Chinese fennels had an appreciable phenolic content, the essential oils from China had better antioxidant property. It is evident that antioxidant activity depends on phytochemical constituents, which in turn is influenced by climatic conditions.

Anti-inflammatory Activity

Type IV allergic reactions, acute, and subacute inflammatory diseases were inhibited by oral administration of methanolic extracts of fruit [79]. Kataoka *et al.*, [80] studied the anti-inflammatory effects of methanolic extract of fennel seeds. The results showed that inflammation was inhibited through cyclooxygenase and lipoxygenase pathways [81]. Mahmoud *et al.* [82], reported a significant increase in plasma level of High-Density Lipoprotein (HDL) cholesterol during an anti-inflammatory activity. On the contrary, it reduced the level of malondialdehyde (MDA) significantly.

The anti-inflammatory action of the ethanolic extracts was studied in Wistar rats and Swiss Albino mice. Analgesic studies were conducted with Albino rats using the formalin test and Albino mice with writhing test. The ethanolic extract produced dosage-dependent inhibition of pain response elicited by acetic acid and formalin. It also induced dosage-dependent inhibition of edema development in the carrageenan-induced inflammation [83]. Özbek [84] reported the anti-inflammatory effect of essential oil that contained (E)-anethole, methyl chavicol, limonene, α-pinene and fenchone on par with etodolac. The blocking of inflammatory processes was through the regulation of pro-inflammatory cytokine production and transcription factors [85].

Analgesic Activity

Any substance that can inhibit the sensation of pain is an antinociceptive substance. The effects of *Foeniculum vulgare* extract in the reduction of pain and other systemic symptoms accompanying primary dysmenorrhea were studied. The severity of pain in the treated group with *Foeniculum vulgare* extract, showed a significant change in systemic symptoms when compared with the placebo group [86].

Acetic acid-induced pain can be due to increased production of prostaglandins and prostacyclins mediated by cyclooxygenases and lipoxygenases [87]. Thus, any phytochemical constituent present in the extract which can inhibit prostaglandin and prostacyclin production through inhibition of cyclooxygenases and lipoxygenases will be able to alleviate such pain. Interestingly, ethanol extract of fruits has inhibited 5- lipoxygenase, which is attributed to the presence of several terpene derivatives including γ-terpinene, fenchone, phenylpropanoid and trans-anethole [88]. Thus, these phytochemicals may account for the observed analgesic activity. Antinociceptive activity was observed in hexane, ethyl acetate, methanol and methylene chloride extracts of aerial part of *F. vulgare* [89]. The highest antinociceptive activity was exhibited by methanol extract, while the other extracts were similar in action with the reference compound acetylsalicylic acid [90].

Antithrombotic and Hepatoprotective Activity

Anethole, an important compound in the essential oil of *F. vulgare* showed antithrombotic activity. Anethole was tested in guinea pig plasma. A positive control was arachidonic acid, collagen-ADP, and U46619 induced aggregation. Anethole was as potent as essential oils in inhibiting aggregation. Anethole also prevented thrombin-induced clotting [91].

The hepatoprotective activity was studied in CCl_4 induced hepatotoxicity. Fennel offered protection against liver toxicity. This was evident by decreased levels of serum alanine aminotransferase (ALT), aspartate aminotransferase (AST), alkaline phosphatase (ALP) and bilirubin [92, 93]. Fennel's effect was also investigated on lipid peroxide in rats with hepatic fibrosis. After oral consumption of fennel, the serum MDA, ALT and AST levels decreased significantly and SOD, CAT, TP, ALB and GSH-PX activities increased. Fennel prevented Hepatic fibrosis by regulating lipid peroxide. Wang *et al.* [94], studied the effect of fennel on cytokines in hepatic fibrotic rats and found fennel treated groups showed a reduction in lipids and inflammation. The above findings indicate that fennel can reduce liver swelling and save hepatocytes significantly.

Antidiabetic Activity

The essential oils showed hypoglycaemic activity in Streptozotocin-induced diabetic rats. Oral administration of diabetic rats with essential oil of *F. vulgare* rectified the hyperglycemia by lowering the activity of serum glutathione peroxidize [95]. Jamshidi *et al.* [96], demonstrated a reduction of blood sugar levels in aqueous fennel extract treatment. Fennel can be very useful for diabetics as it may control the blood sugar levels and reduce the complications associated with diabetes.

Anticancer and Chemomodulatory Action

Cytoprotective activity of methanolic extract of *F. vulgare* was studied on normal human blood lymphocytes. The cryoprotective activity was determined by the percentage of micronuclei formed. Very less micronuclei formation was observed with 70% methanolic extract when compared to standard drug doxorubicin. Methanolic extract exerted remarkable antitumor activity on B16F10 melanoma cell line, liver cancer cell line (Hepg-2) and breast cancer cell line (MCF7) [97, 98]. It exhibits an antitumor effect by modulating lipid peroxidation. This is possible due to the antioxidant property. *Foeniculum vulgare* extracts induced p53 gene expression in cancer cell lines than in untreated cell lines. It showed the differential expression of apoptotic gene (Bax) in cancer cells. There is a direct correlation between gene expression and the number of proteins produced.SDS polyacrylamide gel showed a large number of proteins in fennel treated cancer cell lines when compared to untreated cell lines [99]. Kooti *et al.* [100, 101], found that anethole in fennel seed had an inhibitory effect on the activation of the TNF-α transcription factor. Fennel extract showed cytotoxicity in human breast cancer cell lines. Fennel seeds are a good source of melatonin, which protects against breast cancer by reducing aromatase activity within the breast, thereby reducing estrogen production. Farukh *et al.* [102], also studied the cytotoxic activity of fennel seed extract on Caco-2 (human colorectal adenocarcinoma), MCF-7 (human breast adenocarcinoma), HeLa (human cervical cancer), CEM/ADR5000 (adriamycin resistant leukemia) cancer cell lines and CCRF-CEM (human T lymphoblast leukemia. Low cytotoxicity was observed when compared to reference compounds.

The potential antimutagenic and cancer chemoprevention effects of the hot aqueous crude extract of sweet fennel (*Foeniculum vulgare* Mill.) were studied. The activity was dosage-dependent. However, the RAPD analysis of DNA showed variation between treated and non treated animals. Fennel extracts exerted a protective effect on DNA. In Drosophila, fennel extract significantly decreased the frequency of aneuploidy and chromosomal aberrations induced by colchicine [103]. The apoptotic activity of the crude methanolic extract was investigated in cervical cancer cell lines (HeLa). *Foeniculum vulgare* induced apoptosis and inhibited cell proliferation through DNA fragmentation [104].

The mode of action of anethole was studied on Ehrlich ascites tumor (EAT). Anethole increased the survival rate, reduced body weight, tumor weight, and volume. These effects were due to a reduction in the levels of nucleicacids, which in turn reflected on the frequency of micronuclei and the ratio of polychromatic erythrocytes to normochromic erythrocytes. These findingsrevealed that anethole was mitodepressive and non-clastogenic in nature [105].

Table 1. Phytochemical constituents of *Foeniculum vulgare* with its biological activities.

S. No	Phytochemical	Biological Activity
1	Anethole	Antithrombic [91], Anticancer [99], Antimutagenic [103], Ooestrogenic, Galactogogue [108] and Bronchodilator [83]
2	Phenylpropanoid, Dillapional Scopolitin	Antibacterial activity [46]
3	Fenchone, Limonene, 1,8, Cineole, (E) 9 –Octadecenoic acid, Terpiniol	Antilarvicidal activity [60]
4	Anethole, Limonene	Schistosomicidal activity [66]
5	P-anisaldehyde, thymol, estragole,(+)-fenchone and (-)-fenchone	Ascaricidal activity [64]
6	Quercitin-3-O-galactoside, Kaempferol -3-O-Glucoside, Rosmarinic acid, Estragole, Caffeoylquinic acid Trans-Anethole	Antioxidant activity [22]
7	E-Anethole, Methylchavicol, Limonene, α-pinene, Fenchone	Anti-inflammatory activity [84]
8	γ-terpinene, Fenchone, Phenylpropanoid, Transanethole	Analgesic activity [88]

The chemopreventive effect of fennel seeds was also examined on the skin and stomach papilloma genesis induced by 7,12-dimethylbenz(a)anthracene- (DMBA) and Enzo(a)pyrene-[B(a)P-], respectively. Skin and forestomach tumor incidence and tumor multiplicity reduced when compared to control. Enhanced activities of antioxidant enzymes prove that seeds of fennel are chemopreventive against carcinogenesis [106].

Oestrogenic, Galactogenic and Antihirustism Activities

Phytoestrogens include flavonoids, isoflavonoids, chalcones, coumestans, stilbenes, essential oils, lignans and saponins [107]. *F. vulgare* exhibits estrogen-like activity. On administration of acetone extract in male rats, a significant reduction in the total proteins in testes, vasa deferentia and increased protein in seminal vesicles and prostate glands were evident. Experimental induction of Vaginal cornification and oestrus cycle was carried out in female rats [108]. The oestrogenic activity of fennel was evident when total nucleic acids and protein increased in mammary glands and oviducts. It increased lactation, menstruation, facilitated childbirth and male libido. Polymers of anethole, such as dianethole and photoanethole [109] are the active oestrogenic agent.

Fennel essential oils have an effect on uterine contraction in rats. Dosage dependent activity was observed. It reduced the intensity of oxytocin-induced uterine contraction significantly. Further, no damage was observed in the vital organs of the dead animals [110].

Hirsutism is the occurrence of male pattern hair growth in women who have a normal ovulatory menstrual cycle and serum androgens. It occurs due to disorder in peripheral androgen metabolism. The ethanolic extract of *F. vulgare* is reported to exhibit anti hirsutism activity. Higher concentrations of fennel in topical creams effectively suppressed hirsutism [111].

Foeniculum vulgare is used as a galactagogue substance for a long time [112]. Anethole, an important component of essential oil has structural similarity with Dopamine. Dopamine inhibits prolactin and thereby prevents lactation. Anethole is reported to compete with dopamine and induces prolactin [109]. In young mice, demethylated anethole induces menstruation and formation of lobule alveolar in mammary glands in young female rabbits. The cutaneous application of Anethole increased nipple development in guinea pigs. Recent research has shown that dianethole and photoanethole, polymers of Anethole may be involved in galactogenic activity.

Antiallergic and Anxiolytic Activities

Methanolic extract of *F. vulgare* fruit showed a significant inhibitory effect on delayed hypersensitivity induced by 2,4-dinitrofluorobenzene. The positive effect on immunologically induced swelling suggests the immunosuppressive properties of *F. vulgare* [82]. Anxiety is the feeling of fear and concern resulting in anxiety disorder. Fennel has been used for the treatment of various symptoms of anxiety and its related psychological symptoms. Naga Kishore *et al.* [113], investigated the Anxiolytic activity of ethanolic extract on mice and significant activity was observed.

Antistress and Nootropic Activities

Natural food may serve as an excellent remedy for a number of stress-related disorders [114]. The whole plant extract exhibited notable antistress effects in stress-induced test animals. The antistress activity was evaluated using urinary levels of vanillyl mandelic acid (VMA) and ascorbic acid. The extract elevated the levels of VMA in urine and resulted in excretion of ascorbic acid [115].

Alzheimer's disease is a neurodegenerative disorder associated with the loss of cognitive abilities. One of the characteristic symptoms of Alzheimer's disease is Dementia. Ancient medicine has well-documented evidence for antidepressant activity in fennel. Memory enhancing effect was evident in the whole plant extract. The treated mice showed lesser symptoms of amnesia when compared to the control group. Memory retention and recovery was dosage dependent on the prolonged treatment of the extract [116]. It significantly inhibited acetylcholinesterase in treated mice and hence fennel extracts can be used to treat dementia and Alzheimer's disease [117].

Bronchodilatory Effect

The bronchodilatory effect of fennel was studied. The ciliary motility of the respiratory apparatus was triggered by essential oils of *F. vulgare* seeds. It helps in the expulsion of extraneous corpuscles. The expectoration of mucus, bacteria and other particles was mediated by the contraction of the smooth muscles of the trachea. Hence, it can be used in bronchial and bronchopulmonary disorders [118, 119]. Bronchodilatory action of ethanol and essential oil extracts were reported in guinea pigs. They seem to open the potassium channels, which relaxes the trachea [28]. Moreover, Anethole shares structural similarity with catecholamines, norepinephrine, epinephrine, and dopamine which are responsible for the bronchodilatory effect [83].

Cardiovascular Activity and High Blood Pressure

Sterilized aqueous leaf extract when administered intravenously,significantly reduced the arterial blood pressure without any adverse effect on the heart rate or respiration. Reduced blood pressure may not be mediated through adrenergic, ganglionic, muscarinic or serotonergic receptors [120]. Since fennel seeds are rich in potassium, they flush the excess water from the body through urine. They also reduce the arterial blood pressure without altering the functioning of the heart and change in respiratory rate. The risk of strokes and heart attacks could be effectively managed with the intake of fennel [121, 122]. Diuretic substances promote urine production by the expulsion of sodium. It also reduces the volume of blood in the cardiovascular system. Fennel ethanolic fruit extract is an excellent diuretic agent on par with urea [123]. It had no effect on noradrenaline and hence less effect on arterial vasculature [124].

Hypolipidemic Activity

The aqueous fennel extract showed hypolipidemic activity in Triton WR-1339 induced mice. It resulted in a significant reduction of triglycerides, apolipoprotein-B, and LDL cholesterol. However, there was an evident increase in apolipoprotein A1 and HDL-cholesterol [125].

Anticolitic and Antispasmodic Activity

The Essential oil of fennel regulate contraction of smooth muscles of the trachea and intestine. It is very effective in chronic colitis with gastrointestinal disturbances and blotting of stomach in the case of dyspepsia [126].

The alcoholic extract of fennel along with *Matricaria chamomilla, Rosmarinus officinalis, Melissa officinalis, Carum carvi, Citrus aurantium,* and *Mentha piperita* were tested for antispasmodic activity with acetylcholine and histamine as references. The extract inhibited ileal contractions in guinea pig induced by acetylcholine and histamine [127].

Aqueous extract of *F. vulgare* exhibited antiulcerogenic activity where it significantly reduced the gastric mucosal lesion induced by ethanol in rats. The extract reduced blood malondialdehyde levels and increased ascorbic acid, retinol, nitrite, nitrate and beta-carotene levels [128].

Weight Loss, Antiaging and Osteoporosis

Fennel is known to increase the metabolic rate of sugars and fats in the liver and pancreas by dissolving fat in the bloodstream that can be utilized as an energy source. It can also suppress appetite and help in weight loss [129]. A formulation containing 4% concentrated seed extract of fennel showed significant antiaging effect and moisturized the skin [130].

Postmenopausal osteoporosis can be managed by the intake of fennel, which contains calcium, iron, magnesium, phosphorus, manganese, vitamin K, and zinc, which contribute to the prevention of bone loss. Constituents in fennel are known to reduce osteoclast that mediates the breakage of weakened bones [131].

CONCLUSION

Fennel is one of the popular traditional herb used in a wide range of ethnomedical treatments, especially for abdominal pains, antiemetic, arthritis, cancer, colic in children, conjunctivitis, constipation, depurative, diarrhea, dieresis, emmenagogue, fever, flatulence, gastralgia, gastritis, insomnia, irritable colon, kidney ailments, as a laxative, leucorrhoea, liver pain, mouth ulcer, and stomachache. Numerous studies on *F. vulgare* have shown that it contains innumerable diverse biological properties such as antiaging, antiallergic, anticolitic, antihirsutism, anti-inflammatory, antimicrobial and antiviral, antimutagenic, antinociceptive, antipyretic, antispasmodic, antistress, antithrombotic, anxiolytic, apoptotic, cardiovascular, chemomodulatory action, cytoprotection and antitumor, cytotoxicity, diuretic, estrogenic properties, expectorant, galactogenic, gastrointestinal effect, hepatoprotective, hypoglycemic, hypolipidemic, memory-enhancing property and nootropic supporting its traditional use and yet there are many more to be discovered. Animal and clinical studies have also indicated that the use of fennel has no harmful effect. The phytochemical constituents present in fennel are responsible for the above-mentioned activities. But the reported activities were studied using crude extracts of fennel. There is immense scope and need to characterize, standardize and explore the bioactive compounds. The mechanism of action of many of the bioactive compounds needs to be studied to benefit the society. There is insufficient knowledge on the correlation of geographical distribution, seasonal variation, pharmacognosy, and bioactive compounds. Further research on these aspects will produce more valuable information on *F. vulgare.*

CONSENT FOR PUBLICATION

Not applicable.

CONFLICT OF INTERESTS

The author declares no conflict of interest, financial or otherwise.

ACKNOWLEDGEMENTS

Declared none.

REFERENCES

[1]   Ahmadi A, Nasiri Nejad F, Parivar K. Effect of aqueous extract of the aerial part of the *Ruta graveolens* on the spermatogenesis of immature Balb/C mice. Majallah-i Ulum-i Pizishki-i Razi 2007;

14(56): 13-20.

[2]   Ghaima KK, Hashim NM, Ali SA. Antibacterial and antioxidant activities of ethyl acetate extract of nettle (*Urtica dioica*) and dandelion (*Taraxacum officinale*). J App Pharm Sci 2013; 3(05): 096-9.

[3]   Badgujar SB, Patel VV, Bandivdekar AH. *Foeniculum vulgare* Mill: a review of its botany, phytochemistry, pharmacology, contemporary application, and toxicology. BioMed Res Int 2014; 2014842674
[http://dx.doi.org/10.1155/2014/842674] [PMID: 25162032]

[4]   Xue GQ, Liu Q, Han YQ, Wei HG, Dong T. Determination of thirteen metal elements in the plant *Foeniculum vulgare* Mill. by flame atomic absorption spectrophotometry. Guangpuxue Yu Guangpu Fenxi 2006; 26(10): 1935-8.
[PMID: 17205757]

[5]   Díaz-Maroto MC, Pérez-Coello MS, Esteban J, Sanz J. Comparison of the volatile composition of wild fennel samples (*Foeniculum vulgare* Mill.) from central Spain. J Agric Food Chem 2006; 54(18): 6814-8.
[http://dx.doi.org/10.1021/jf0609532] [PMID: 16939344]

[6]   The plant list, a working list of all plant species, Foeniculum vulgare Mill http://ipni.org/urn:lsid: Ipni.org:names;842680-1.

[7]   Endalamaw FD, Chandravanshi BS. Levels of major and trace elements in fennel (*Foeniculum vulgare* Mill.) fruits cultivated in Ethiopia. Springerplus 2015; 4: 5.
[http://dx.doi.org/10.1186/2193-1801-4-5] [PMID: 25674492]

[8]   Gori L, Gallo E, Mascherini V, Mugelli A, Vannacci A, Firenzuoli F. Can estragole in fennel seed decoctions really be considered a danger for human health? A fennel safety update. Evid Based Complement Alternat Med 2012; 2012860542
[http://dx.doi.org/10.1155/2012/860542] [PMID: 22899959]

[9]   Taherian A, Dehghanina M, Vafaei AA, Sadeghi H, Miladi Gorgi H. Effects of aqueous extract of fruit of Foeniculum vulgar on neurogenic and inflammatory pain in mice. Majallah-i Ilmi-i Danishgah-i Ulum-i Pizishki-i Kurdistan 2007; 12(2): 29-36.

[10]   Jarić S, Mitrović M, Djurdjević L, *et al.* Phytotherapy in medieval Serbian medicine according to the pharmacological manuscripts of the Chilandar Medical Codex (15-16th centuries). J Ethnopharmacol 2011; 137(1): 601-19.
[http://dx.doi.org/10.1016/j.jep.2011.06.016] [PMID: 21708242]

[11]   Hsu Hong-Yen. Peacher WG Chinese Herb Medicine and Therapy. Oriental Healing Art Institute 1976; p. 172.

[12]   Agarwal R, Gupta SK, Agarwal SS, Srivastava S, Saxena R. Oculohypotensive effects of *Foeniculum vulgare* in experimental models of glaucoma. Indian J Physiol pharmacol 2008; 52: 77-83.

[13]   Osol A, Pratt R, Altschule MD. The United States Dispensatory and Physicians Pharmacology. 26th ed., Philadelphia: J B Lippincott Co. 1960.

[14]   Ramstad E. Modern Pharmacognosy. New York: Mc Graw Hill Book Co. Inc. 1959; p. 480.

[15]   Raal A, Orav A, Arak E. Essential oil composition of *Foeniculum vulgare* Mill. fruits from pharmacies in different countries. Nat Prod Res 2012; 26(13): 1173-8.
[http://dx.doi.org/10.1080/14786419.2010.535154] [PMID: 21827282]

[16]   De Marino S, Gala F, Borbone N, *et al.* Phenolic glycosides from *Foeniculum vulgare* fruit and evaluation of antioxidative activity. Phytochemistry 2007; 68(13): 1805-12.
[http://dx.doi.org/10.1016/j.phytochem.2007.03.029] [PMID: 17498761]

[17]   Barros L, Heleno SA, Carvalho AM, Ferreira IC. Systematic evaluation of the antioxidant potential of different parts of *Foeniculumvulgare* Mill. from Portugal. Food Chem Toxicol 2009; 47(10): 2458-64.
[http://dx.doi.org/10.1016/j.fct.2009.07.003] [PMID: 19596397]

[18]   Jeambey Z, Johns T, Talhouk S, Batal M. Perceived health and medicinal properties of six species of wild edible plants in north-east Lebanon. Public Health Nutr 2009; 12(10): 1902-11.
[http://dx.doi.org/10.1017/S1368980009004832] [PMID: 19232151]

[19]   Robert DA, Shirley ML, Juliett C. Medicinal Plants of the Guianas. Guyana, Surinam, French Guiana 2004; p. 17.

[20]   Kokwaro JO. Medicinal Plants of East Africa. East African Literature Bureau.: Kampala, Nairobi, Dar es Salam 1976.

[21]   Manzoor AR, Dar BA, Sofi NS, Bhat BA, Qurishi MA. *Foeniculum vulgare*: A comprehensive review of its traditional use, phytochemistry, Pharmacology and safety. Arab J Chem 2016; 9(2): S1574-83.

[22]   Musharaf K, Shahana M. Foeniculum vulgare. Mill. A Medicinal Herb 2014; p. 842674.

[23]   Díaz-Maroto MC, Díaz-Maroto Hidalgo IJ, Sánchez-Palomo E, Pérez-Coello MS. Volatile components and key odorants of fennel (*Foeniculum vulgare* Mill.) and thyme (Thymus vulgaris L.) oil extracts obtained by simultaneous distillation-extraction and supercritical fluid extraction. J Agric Food Chem 2005; 53(13): 5385-9.
[http://dx.doi.org/10.1021/jf050340+] [PMID: 15969523]

[24]   Meireles MA. Supercritical fluid extraction from fennel (*Foeniculum vulgare*): global yield, composition and kinetic data. J Supercrit Fluids 2005; 35(3): 212-9.
[http://dx.doi.org/10.1016/j.supflu.2005.01.006]

[25]   Rather MA, Dar BA, Sofi SN, Bhat BA, Qurishi MA. *Foeniculum vulgare*: A comprehensive review of its traditional use, phytochemistry, pharmacology, and safety. Arab J Chem 2012.

[26]   Miguel MG, Cruz C, Faleiro L, *et al. Foeniculum vulgare* essential oils: chemical composition, antioxidant and antimicrobial activities. Nat Prod Commun 2010; 5(2): 319-28.
[http://dx.doi.org/10.1177/1934578X1000500231] [PMID: 20334152]

[27]   Salehi Surmaghi H. Medicinal plants and phytotherapy. Tehran, Iran: Donyaee Taghazie 2006; pp. 59-63.

[28]   Rahimi R, Ardekani MRS. Medicinal properties of *Foeniculum vulgare* Mill. in traditional Iranian medicine and modern phytotherapy. Chin J Integr Med 2013; 19(1): 73-9.
[http://dx.doi.org/10.1007/s11655-013-1327-0] [PMID: 23275017]

[29]   Bagdassarian Christova VL, Bagdassarian KS. Phenolic profile, antioxidant and antimicrobial activities from the Apiaceae family (dryseeds) Mintag. Journal of Pharmaceutical&Medical Sciences 2013; 2(4): 26-31.

[30]   Faudale M, Viladomat F, Bastida J, Poli F, Codina C. Antioxidant activity and phenolic composition of wild, edible, and medicinal fennel from different Mediterranean countries. J Agric Food Chem 2008; 56(6): 1912-20.
[http://dx.doi.org/10.1021/jf073083c] [PMID: 18303817]

[31]   Parejo I, Jauregui O, Sánchez-Rabaneda F, Viladomat F, Bastida J, Codina C. Separation and characterization of phenolic compounds in fennel (*Foeniculum vulgare*) using liquid chromatography-negative electrospray ionization tandem mass spectrometry. J Agric Food Chem 2004; 52(12): 3679-87.
[http://dx.doi.org/10.1021/jf030813h] [PMID: 15186082]

[32]   Abed KF. Antimicrobial activity of essential oils of some medicinal plants from Saudi Arabia. Saudi J Biol Sci 2007; 14: 53-60.

[33]   Fennel (*Foeniculum vulgare* Mill.): A Common Spice with Unique Medicinal Properties. Annals of Complementary and Alternative Medicine 2018; 1(1): 1-9.

[34]   Kaur GJ, Arora DS. Antibacterial and phytochemical screening of *Anethum graveolens, Foeniculum vulgare* and *Trachyspermum ammi*. BMC Complement Altern Med 2009; 9: 30.
[http://dx.doi.org/10.1186/1472-6882-9-30] [PMID: 19656417]

[35]   Mahady GB, Pendland SL, Stoia A, *et al. In vitro* susceptibility of *Helicobacter pylori* to botanical extracts used traditionally for the treatment of gastrointestinal disorders. Phytother Res 2005; 19(11): 988-91.
[http://dx.doi.org/10.1002/ptr.1776] [PMID: 16317658]

[36]   Yaralizadeh M, Abedi P, Najar S, Namjoyan F, Saki A. Effect of *Foeniculum vulgare* (fennel) vaginal cream on vaginal atrophy in postmenopausal women: A double-blind randomized placebo-controlled trial. Maturitas 2016; 84: 75-80.
[http://dx.doi.org/10.1016/j.maturitas.2015.11.005] [PMID: 26617271]

[37]   Akha O, Rabiei K, Kashi Z, *et al.* The effect of fennel (*Foeniculum vulgare*) gel 3% in decreasing hair thickness in idiopathic mild to moderate hirsutism, A randomized placebo controlled clinical trial. Caspian J Intern Med 2014; 5(1): 26-9.
[PMID: 24490010]

[38]   Mohsenzadeh M. Evaluation of antibacterial activity of selected Iranian essential oils against Staphylococcus aureus and Escherichia coli in nutrient broth medium. Pak J Biol Sci 2007; 10(20): 3693-7.
[http://dx.doi.org/10.3923/pjbs.2007.3693.3697] [PMID: 19093484]

[39]   Dadalioglu I, Evrendilek GA. Chemical compositions and antibacterial effects of essential oils of Turkish oregano (*Origanum minutiflorum*), bay laurel (*Laurus nobilis*), Spanish lavender (*Lavandula stoechas* L.), and fennel (*Foeniculum vulgare*) on common foodborne pathogens. J Agric Food Chem 2004; 52: 8255-60.

[40]   Mota AS, Martins MR, Arantes S, *et al.* Antimicrobial activity and chemical composition of the essential oils of Portuguese *Foeniculum vulgare* fruits. Nat Prod Commun 2015; 10(4): 673-6.
[http://dx.doi.org/10.1177/1934578X1501000437] [PMID: 25973507]

[41]   Aprotosoaie AC, Hăncianu M, Poiată A, *et al. In vitro* antimicrobial activity and chemical composition of the essential oil of *Foeniculum vulgare* Mill. Rev Med Chir Soc Med Nat Iasi 2008; 112(3): 832-6.
[PMID: 20201277]

[42]   Lixandru BE, Drăcea NO, Dragomirescu CC, *et al.* Antimicrobial activity of plant essential oils against bacterial and fungal species involved in food poisoning and/or food decay. Roum Arch Microbiol Immunol 2010; 69(4): 224-30.
[PMID: 21462837]

[43]   Jazani NH, Zartoshti M, Babazadeh H, Ali-daiee N, Zarrin S, Hosseini S. Antibacterial effects of Iranian fennel essential oil on isolates of *Acinetobacter baumannii*. Pak J Biol Sci 2009; 12(9): 738-41.
[http://dx.doi.org/10.3923/pjbs.2009.738.741] [PMID: 19634482]

[44]   Cwikla C, Schmidt K, Matthias A, Bone KM, Lehmann R, Tiralongo E. Investigations into the antibacterial activities of phytotherapeutics against *Helicobacter pylori* and *Campylobacter jejuni*. Phytother Res 2010; 24(5): 649-56.
[PMID: 19653313]

[45]   Camacho-Corona MdelR, Ramírez-Cabrera MA, Santiago OG, Garza-González E, Palacios IdeP, Luna-Herrera J. Activity against drug resistant-tuberculosis strains of plants used in Mexican traditional medicine to treat tuberculosis and other respiratory diseases. Phytother Res 2008; 22(1): 82-5.
[http://dx.doi.org/10.1002/ptr.2269] [PMID: 17726732]

[46]   Qiu J, Li H, Su H, *et al.* Chemical composition of fennel essential oil and its impact on *Staphylococcus aureus* exotoxin production. World J Microbiol Biotechnol 2012; 28(4): 1399-405.
[http://dx.doi.org/10.1007/s11274-011-0939-4] [PMID: 22805920]

[47]   Pecarski D, Dragićević-Ćurić N, Jugović Z. Chemical composition, antifungal and antibacterial potential of fennel (*Foeniculum vulgare*) and cumin (Carum carvi) essential oils (Apiaceae). Rastenievadni nauki. Rastenievudni Nauki 2017; 54(1): 66-72.

[48]　Neetu T. Studies on *In vitro* antifungal activity of *Foeniculum vulgare* mill. against spoilage fungi GJBB 2013; 2(3): 427-30.

[49]　Aaamir F, Bashir H, Mahmood M. Antifungal Activity of Freshly Growing Seeds of Fennel (*Foeniculum vulgare*). P J M H S 2018; 12(4): 1487-8.

[50]　Samah AAR, Elamin BEK, Bashir AAA, Almagboul AZ. In *Vitro* Test Of Antimicrobial Activity Of *Foeniculum Vulgare* Mill. (Fennel) Essential Oil. Journal of Multidisciplinary Engineering Science Studies 2017; 3(4): 1609-14.

[51]　Shahat AA, Ibrahim AY, Hendawy SF, *et al.* Chemical composition, antimicrobial and antioxidant activities of essential oils from organically cultivated fennel cultivars. Molecules 2011; 16(2): 1366-77.
[http://dx.doi.org/10.3390/molecules16021366] [PMID: 21285921]

[52]　Pai MB, Prashant GM, Murlikrishna KS, Shivakumar KM, Chandu GN. Antifungal efficacy of *Punica granatum, Acacia nilotica, Cuminum cyminum* and *Foeniculum vulgare* on *Candida albicans*: an *In vitro* study. Indian J Dent Res 2010; 21(3): 334-6.
[http://dx.doi.org/10.4103/0970-9290.70792] [PMID: 20930339]

[53]　Alizadeh A, Zamani E, Sharaifi R, Javan-Nikkhah M, Nazari S. Antifungal activity of some essential oils against toxigenic *Aspergillus* species. Commun Agric Appl Biol Sci 2010; 75(4): 761-7.
[PMID: 21534488]

[54]　Zeng H, Chen X, Liang J. *In vitro* antifungal activity and mechanism of essential oil from fennel (*Foeniculum vulgare* L.) on dermatophyte species. J Med Microbiol 2015; 64(Pt 1): 93-103.
[http://dx.doi.org/10.1099/jmm.0.077768-0] [PMID: 25351709]

[55]　Soylu S, Yigitbas H, Soylu EM, Kurt S. Antifungal effects of essential oils from oregano and fennel on *Sclerotinia sclerotiorum*. J Appl Microbiol 2007; 103: 1021-30.

[56]　Singh G, Maurya S, de Lampasona MP, Catalan C. Chemical constituents, antifungal and antioxidative potential of Foeniculum vulgare volatile oil and its acetone extract. Food Control 2006; 17: 745-52.
[http://dx.doi.org/10.1016/j.foodcont.2005.03.010]

[57]　Orhan I, Kartal M, Kan Y, Sener B. Activity of essential oils and individual components against acetyl- and butyrylcholinesterase. Z Natforsch C J Biosci 2008; 63(7-8): 547-53.
[http://dx.doi.org/10.1515/znc-2008-7-813] [PMID: 18810999]

[58]　Kim DH, Kim SI, Chang KS, Ahn YJ. Repellent activity of constituents identified in *Foeniculum vulgare* fruit against *Aedes aegypti* (Diptera: Culicidae). J Agric Food Chem 2002; 50(24): 6993-6.
[http://dx.doi.org/10.1021/jf020504b] [PMID: 12428949]

[59]　Zoubiri S, Baaliouamer A, Seba N, Chamoun N. Chemical composition and larvicidal activity of Algerian *Foeniculum vulgare* seed essential oil. Arab J Chem 2014; 7: 480-5.
[http://dx.doi.org/10.1016/j.arabjc.2010.11.006]

[60]　Rocha DK, Matosc O, Novoa MT, Figueiredo AC, Delgado M, Moiteiro C. Larvicidal activity against *Aedes aegypti* of *Foeniculum vulgare* essential oils from Portugal and Cape Verde. Nat Prod Commun 2015; 10(4): 677-82.
[http://dx.doi.org/10.1177/1934578X1501000438] [PMID: 25973508]

[61]　Sedaghat MM, Sanei Dehkordi A, Abai MR. Larvicidal activity of essential oils of apiaceae plants against malaria vector, *Anopheles stephensi*. Journal of Arthropod-Borne Diseases 2011.

[62]　Traboulsi AF, El-Haj S, Tueni M, Taoubi K, Nader NA, Mrad A. Repellency and toxicity of aromatic plant extracts against the mosquito *Culex pipiens molestus* (Diptera: Culicidae). Pest Manag Sci 2005; 61(6): 597-604.
[http://dx.doi.org/10.1002/ps.1017] [PMID: 15662650]

[63]　Abbas B, Al-Qarawi AA, Al-Hawas A. The ethnoveterinary knowledge and practice of traditional healers in Qassim Region, Saudi Arabia. J Arid Environ 2002; 50: 367-79.

[http://dx.doi.org/10.1006/jare.2001.0904]

[64]   Lee HS. Acaricidal activity of constituents identified in *Foeniculum vulgare* fruit oil against Dermatophagoides spp. (Acari: Pyroglyphidae). J Agric Food Chem 2004; 52(10): 2887-9.
[http://dx.doi.org/10.1021/jf049631t] [PMID: 15137830]

[65]   Study of antibacterial, antimycobacterial antifungal, and antioxidant activities of Foeniculum vulgare: A review 2 Der Pharmacia Lettre 2016; 8(9): 200-5.

[66]   Wakabayashi KA, de Melo NI, Aguiar DP, *et al.* Anthelmintic effects of the essential oil of fennel (*Foeniculum vulgare* Mill., Apiaceae) against Schistosoma mansoni. Chem Biodivers 2015; 12(7): 1105-14.
[http://dx.doi.org/10.1002/cbdv.201400293] [PMID: 26172330]

[67]   Oka Y, Nacar S, Putievsky E, Ravid U, Yaniv Z, Spiegel Y. Nematicidal activity of essential oils and their components against the root-knot nematode. Phytopathology 2000; 90(7): 710-5.
[http://dx.doi.org/10.1094/PHYTO.2000.90.7.710] [PMID: 18944489]

[68]   Sokkar NM, Ali ZY, Yehia MM. A profile of bioactive compounds of *Rumex vesicarius*L. J Food Sci 2012; 76: 1195-202.

[69]   Cieslik EA. Greda, W. Adamus, Contents of polyphenols in fruits and vegetables. Food Chem 2006; 52: 135-42.
[http://dx.doi.org/10.1016/j.foodchem.2004.11.015]

[70]   Goswami N, Chatterjee S. Assessment of free radical scavenging potential and oxidative DNA damage preventive activity of *Trachyspermum ammi* L. (carom) and *Foeniculum vulgare* Mill. (fennel) seed extracts. BioMed Res Int 2014; 2014582767
[http://dx.doi.org/10.1155/2014/582767] [PMID: 25143939]

[71]   Mohamad RH, El-Bastawesy AM, Abdel-Monem MG, Noor AM. Al- Mehdar HA, Sharawy SM. Antioxidant and anti-carcinogenic effects of methanolic extract and volatile oil of fennel seeds (*Foeniculum vulgare*). J Med Food 2011; 14(9): 986-1001.
[http://dx.doi.org/10.1089/jmf.2008.0255] [PMID: 21812646]

[72]   Parejo I, Viladomat F, Bastida J, *et al.* Comparison between the radical scavenging activity and antioxidant activity of six distilled and nondistilled mediterranean herbs and aromatic plants. J Agric Food Chem 2002; 50(23): 6882-90.
[http://dx.doi.org/10.1021/jf020540a] [PMID: 12405792]

[73]   Yang IJ, Lee DU, Shin HM. Anti-inflammatory and antioxidant effects of coumarins isolated from *Foeniculum vulgare* in lipopolysaccharide-stimulated macrophages and 12-O-tetradecanoylphorb-l-13-acetate-stimulated mice. Immunopharmacol Immunotoxicol 2015; 37(3): 308-17.
[http://dx.doi.org/10.3109/08923973.2015.1038751] [PMID: 25990850]

[74]   Satyanarayana S, Sushruta K, Sarma GS, Srinivas N, Subba Raju GV. Antioxidant activity of the aqueous extracts of spicy food additives--evaluation and comparison with ascorbic acid in in-vitro systems. J Herb Pharmacother 2004; 4(2): 1-10.
[http://dx.doi.org/10.1080/J157v04n02_01] [PMID: 15364640]

[75]   Papageorgiou V, Mallouchos A, Komaitis M. Investigation of the antioxidant behavior of air- and freeze-dried aromatic plant materials in relation to their phenolic content and vegetative cycle. J Agric Food Chem 2008; 56(14): 5743-52.
[http://dx.doi.org/10.1021/jf8009393] [PMID: 18578534]

[76]   Guimarães R, Barreira JC, Barros L, Carvalho AM, Ferreira IC. Effects of oral dosage form and storage period on the antioxidant properties of four species used in traditional herbal medicine. Phytother Res 2011; 25(4): 484-92.
[http://dx.doi.org/10.1002/ptr.3284] [PMID: 20740475]

[77]   De Marino S, Gala F, Borbone N, *et al.* Phenolic glycosides from *Foeniculum vulgare* fruit and evaluation of antioxidative activity. Phytochemistry 2007; 68(13): 1805-12.

[http://dx.doi.org/10.1016/j.phytochem.2007.03.029] [PMID: 17498761]

[78] Ahmed AF, Shib MC, Liub C, Wenyi K. Comparative analysis of antioxidant activities of essential oils and extracts of fennel (*Foeniculum vulgare* Mill.) seeds from Egypt and China. Food Sci Hum Wellness 2019; 8(1): 67-72.
[http://dx.doi.org/10.1016/j.fshw.2019.03.004]

[79] Choi EM, Hwang JK. Antiinflammatory, analgesic and antioxidant activities of the fruit of *Foeniculum vulgare.* Fitoterapia 2004; 75(6): 557-65.
[http://dx.doi.org/10.1016/j.fitote.2004.05.005] [PMID: 15351109]

[80] Kataoka H, Horiyama S, Yamaki M, *et al.* Anti-inflammatory and anti-allergic activities of hydroxylamine and related compounds. Biol Pharm Bull 2002; 25(11): 1436-41.
[http://dx.doi.org/10.1248/bpb.25.1436] [PMID: 12419955]

[81] Albert-Puleo M. Fennel and anise as estrogenic agents. J Ethnopharmacol 1980; 2(4): 337-44.
[http://dx.doi.org/10.1016/S0378-8741(80)81015-4] [PMID: 6999244]

[82] Nasser MI. Sayed EL, Aboutabl A, Makled YA. Secondary metabolites and pharmacology of *Foeniculum vulgare* mill. J Pharmacogn Phytochem 2010; 28(2): 220.

[83] Elizabeth AA, Josephine G, Muthiah NS, Muniappan M. Evaluation of analgesic and anti-inflammatory effect of *Foeniculum vulgare.* Res J Pharm Biol Chem Sci 2014; 5(2): 658-68.

[84] Özbek H. The anti-inflammatory activity of the *Foeniculum vulgare* L. essential oil and Investigationof its Medium lethal dose in rats and mice. Int J Pharmacol 2005; 1(4): 329-31.
[http://dx.doi.org/10.3923/ijp.2005.329.331]

[85] Lee HS, Kang P, Kim KY, Seol GH. *Foeniculum vulgare* Mill. Protects against lipopolysaccharide-induced acute lung injury in mice through ERK-dependent NF-κB activation. Korean J Physiol Pharmacol 2015; 19(2): 183-9.
[http://dx.doi.org/10.4196/kjpp.2015.19.2.183] [PMID: 25729281]

[86] Torkzahrani SH, Amjadi AM, Mojab F, Alavimajd H. Clinical effects of *Foeniculum vulgare* extract on primary dysmenorrhea. J Reprod Infertil 2007; 8(1): 45-51.

[87] Taherian A, Dehghanina M, Vafaei AA, Sadeghi H, Miladi Gorgi H. Effects of aqueous extract of fruit of *Foeniculum vulgae* on neurogenic and inflammatory pain in mice. Majallah-i Ilmi-i Danishgah-i Ulum-i Pizishki-i Kurdistan 2007; 12(2): 29-36.

[88] Lee JH, Lee DU, Kim YS, Kim HP. 5-Lipoxygenase Inhibition of the Fructus of Foeniculum vulgare and Its Constituents. Biomol Ther (Seoul) 2012; 20(1): 113-7.
[http://dx.doi.org/10.4062/biomolther.2012.20.1.113] [PMID: 24116283]

[89] Nassar MI, Aboutabl EA, Makled YA, ElKhrisy EA, Osman AF. Secondary metabolites and pharmacology of *Foeniculum vulgare* Mill. Subsp. *Piperitum.* Rev Latinoam Quím 2010; 38(2): 103-12.

[90] Shanmugasundaram P, Venkataraman S. Anti nociceptive activity of Hygrophilous auriculata (Schum) Heine. Afr J Tradit Complement Altern Med 2005; 2(1): 62-9.

[91] Tognolini M, Ballabeni V, Bertoni S, Bruni R, Impicciatore M, Barocelli E. Protective effect of *Foeniculum vulgare* essential oil and anethole in an experimental model of thrombosis. Pharmacol Res 2007; 56(3): 254-60.
[http://dx.doi.org/10.1016/j.phrs.2007.07.002] [PMID: 17709257]

[92] Ozbek H, U˘gras S˛. Hepatoprotective effect of *Foeniculum vulgare* essential oil. Fitoterapia 2003; 74(3): 317-9.

[93] Qiang F, Yiming A, Shui-quan W, Zi-ming G. Effects of *Foeniculum vulgare* Mill on lipid peroxidation in rats with liver hepatic fibrosis. Prog Mod Biomed 2011; 21: 13.

[94] Wang L, Zhang T, Zhang JL. YU Y, Gan ZM. Experimental study of Chinese herb *Foeniculum vulgare* Mill on liver hepatic fibrosis and potassiumsupplement in rats. Xinjiang Yike Daxue Xuebao

2012; 9: 12.

[95] El-Soud NA, El-Laithy N, El-Saeed G. Antidiabetic activities of *Foeniculum vulgare* mill. Essentialoil in streptozotocin-induced diabetic rats. Maced J Med Sci 2011; 4(2): 139-46.

[96] Jamshidi E, Ghalavand A, Sefidkon F, Goltaph E. Effects of different nutrition systems (organic and chemical) on quantitative and qualitative characteristics of Fennel (*Foeniculum vulgare* Mill.) under water deficit stress. Tahqiqat-i Giyahan-i Daruyi va Muattar-i Iran 2012; 28(2): 309-23.

[97] Pradhan M, Sribhuwaneswari S, Karthikeyan D. *In-vitro* cytoprotection activity of *Foeniculum vulgare* and *Helicteres isora* in cultured human blood lymphocytes and antitumour activity against B16F10 melanoma cell line. Research Journal of Pharmacy and Technology 2008; 1(4): 450-2.

[98] Mohamad RH, El-Bastawesy AM, Abdel-Monem MG, *et al.* Antioxidant and anticarcinogenic effects of methanolic extract and volatile oil of fennel seeds (*Foeniculum vulgare*). J Med Food 2011; 14(9): 986-1001.
[http://dx.doi.org/10.1089/jmf.2008.0255] [PMID: 21812646]

[99] Samir AM. Zaahkouk, Ezzat. Aboul-Ela, Ramadan MA, Sayed Bakry and Ahmed BM. Anticarcinogenic activity of Methanolic Extract of Fennel Seeds (*Foeniculum vulgare*) against breast,colon, and liver cancer cells. Int J Adv Res (Indore) 2015; 3(5): 1525-37.

[100] Kooti W, Mansouri E, Ghasemiboroon M, Harizi M, Ashtary-Larky D, Afrisham R. The Effects of hydroalcoholic extract of apium grave lens leaf on the number of sexual cells and testicular structure in rat. Jundishapur J Nat Pharm Prod 2014; 9(4)e17532
[http://dx.doi.org/10.17795/jjnpp-17532] [PMID: 25625050]

[101] Kooti W, Ghasemiboroon M, Asadi-Samani M, Ahangarpoor A, Abadi A. The effects of hydro-alcoholic extract of celery on lipid profile of rats fed a high fat diet. Adv Environ Biol 2014; 8(9): 325-30.

[102] Sharopov F, Valiev A, Satyal P, *et al.* Cytotoxicity of the Essential Oil of Fennel (*Foeniculum vulgare*) from Tajikistan. Foods 2017; 6(9): 73.
[http://dx.doi.org/10.3390/foods6090073] [PMID: 28846628]

[103] Ebeed NM, Abdou HS, Booles HF, Salah SH, Ahmed ES, Fahmy KH. Antimutagenic and chemoprevention potentialities of sweet fennel *(Foeniculum vulgare* Mill.) hot water crude extract. J Am Sci 2010; 6(9): 831-42.

[104] Devika V, Mohandass S. Apoptotic induction of crude extract of *Foeniculum vulgare* extracts on cervical cancer cell lines. Int J Curr Microbiol Appl Sci 2014; 3(3): 657-61.

[105] al-Harbi MM, Qureshi S, Raza M, Ahmed MM, Giangreco AB, Shah AH. Influence of anethole treatment on the tumour induced by Ehrlich ascites carcinoma cells in paw of Swiss albino mice. Eur J Cancer Prev 1995; 4(4): 307-18.
[http://dx.doi.org/10.1097/00008469-199508000-00006] [PMID: 7549823]

[106] Birdane FM, Cemek M, Birdane YO, Gülçin I, Büyükokuroğlu ME. Beneficial effects of *Foeniculum vulgare* on ethanol-induced acute gastric mucosal injury in rats. World J Gastroenterol 2007; 13(4): 607-11.
[http://dx.doi.org/10.3748/wjg.v13.i4.607] [PMID: 17278229]

[107] He W, Huang B. A review of chemistry and bioactivities of a medicinal spice: *Foeniculum vulgare*. J Med Plants Res 2011; 5(16): 3595-600.

[108] Devi K, Vanithakumari G, Anusya S, Mekala N, Malini T, Elango V. Effect of *foeniculum vulgare* seed extract on mammary glands and oviducts of ovariectomised rats. Anc Sci Life 1985; 5(2): 129-32.
[PMID: 22557513]

[109] Javidnia K, Dastgheib L, Mohammadi Samani S, Nasiri A. Antihirsutism activity of Fennel (fruits of Foeniculum vulgare) extract. A double-blind placebo controlled study. Phytomedicine 2003; 10(6-7): 455-8.

[http://dx.doi.org/10.1078/094471103322331386] [PMID: 13678227]

[110] Ostad SN, Soodi M, Shariffzadeh M, Khorshidi N, Marzban H. The effect of fennel essential oil on uterine contraction as a model for dysmenorrhea, pharmacology and toxicology study. J Ethnopharmacol 2001; 76(3): 299-304.
[http://dx.doi.org/10.1016/S0378-8741(01)00249-5] [PMID: 11448553]

[111] Malini T, Vanithakumari G. Effect of *Foeniculum vulgare*. Mill seed extract on the genital organs of male and female rats. Indian Journal of Physiology and Pharmacology 1985; 29(1): 21-6.

[112] Müller-Limmroth W, Fröhlich HH. Effect of various phytotherapeutic expectorants on mucociliary transport. Fortschr Med 1980; 98(3): 95-101.
[PMID: 7364365]

[113] Naga Kishore RN, Anjaneyulu M. Naga Ganesh, and Sravya N. Evaluation of anxiolytic activity of ethanolic extract of *Foeniculum vulgare* in mice model. Int J Pharm Pharm Sci 2012; 4(3): 584-6.

[114] Padma P, Khosa RL. Anti-stress agents from natural origin. J Nat Rem 2002; 2(1): 21-7.

[115] *Foeniculum vulgare* Mill (Umbelliferae) attenuates stress and improves memory in wister rats. Trop J Pharm Res 2013; 12(4): 553-8.

[116] Joshi H, Parle M. Cholinergic basis of memory-strengthening effect of *Foeniculum vulgare* Linn. J Med Food 2006; 9(3): 413-7.
[http://dx.doi.org/10.1089/jmf.2006.9.413] [PMID: 17004908]

[117] Lim, Edible Medicinal and Non-Medicinal Plants. NewYork, NY, USA: Springer 2013; Vol. 5.

[118] Reiter M, Brandt W. Relaxant effects on tracheal and ileal smooth muscles of the guinea pig. Arzneimittelforschung 1985; 35(1A): 408-14.
[PMID: 4039178]

[119] Boskabady MH, Khatami A, Nazari A. Possible mechanism(s) for relaxant effects of *Foeniculum vulgare* on guinea pig tracheal chains. Pharmazie 2004; 59(7): 561-4.
[PMID: 15296096]

[120] El Bardai S, Lyoussi B, Wibo M, Morel N. Pharmacological evidence of hypotensive activity of *Marrubium vulgare* and *Foeniculum vulgare* in spontaneously hypertensive rat. Clin Exp Hypertens 2001; 23(4): 329-43.
[http://dx.doi.org/10.1081/CEH-100102671] [PMID: 11349824]

[121] Forster HB, Niklas H, Lutz S. Antispasmodic effects of some medicinal plants. Planta Med 1980; 40(4): 309-19.
[http://dx.doi.org/10.1055/s-2008-1074977] [PMID: 7220648]

[122] Beaux D, Fleurentin J, Mortier F. Diuretic action of hydroalcohol extracts of *Foeniculum vulgare* var dulce (D.C.) roots in rat. Phytother Res 1997; 11: 320-2.
[http://dx.doi.org/10.1002/(SICI)1099-1573(199706)11:4<320::AID-PTR92>3.0.CO;2-N]

[123] Tanira MO, Shah AH, Mohsin A, Ageel AM, Qureshi S. Pharmacological and toxicological investigations on *Foeniculum vulgare* dried fruit extract in experimental animals. Phytother Res 1996; 10(1): 33-6.
[http://dx.doi.org/10.1002/(SICI)1099-1573(199602)10:1<33::AID-PTR769>3.0.CO;2-L]

[124] Cáceres A, Girón LM, Martínez AM. Diuretic activity of plants used for the treatment of urinary ailments in Guatemala. J Ethnopharmacol 1987; 19(3): 233-45.
[http://dx.doi.org/10.1016/0378-8741(87)90001-8] [PMID: 3669686]

[125] Oulmouden F, Saïle R, El Gnaoui N, Benomar H, Lkhider M. Hypolipidemic and anti- atherogenic effect of aqueous extract of fennel (*Foeniculum vulgare*) extract in an experimental model of atherosclerosis induced by Triton WR-1339. Eur J Sci Res 2011; 52(1): 91-9.

[126] Chakŭrski I, Matev M, Koĭchev A, Angelova I, Stefanov G. [Treatment of chronic colitis with an herbal combination of *Taraxacum officinale*, *Hipericum perforatum*, *Melissa officinaliss*, *Calendula*

officinalis and *Foeniculum vulgare*]. Vutr Boles 1981; 20(6): 51-4.
[PMID: 7336706]

[127] Abdul-Ghani AS, Amin R. The vascular action of aqueous extracts of *Foeniculum vulgare* Leaves. Journal of Ethnopharmacology 1988; 24(2-3): 213-8.

[128] Singh B, Kale RK. Chemomodulatory action of *Foeniculum vulgare* (Fennel) on skin and forestomach papillomagenesis, enzymes associated with xenobiotic metabolism and antioxidant status in murine model system. Food Chem Toxicol 2008; 46(12): 3842-50.
[http://dx.doi.org/10.1016/j.fct.2008.10.008] [PMID: 18976688]

[129] Garg C, Ansari SH, Khan SA, Garg M. Effect of *Foeniculum vulgare* mill. fruits in obesity and associated cardiovascular disorders demonstrated in high fat diet fed albino rats. J Pharm Biomed Sci 2011; 8(19): 1-5.

[130] Rasul A, Akhtar N, Khan BA, Mahmood T, Uz Zaman S, Khan HM. Formulation development of a cream containing fennel extract: *in vivo* evaluation for anti-aging effects. Pharmazie 2012; 67(1): 54-8.
[PMID: 22393831]

[131] Mahmoudi Z, Soleimani M, Saidi A, Khamisipour G, Azizsoltani A. Effects of *Foeniculum vulgare* ethanol extract on osteogenesis in human mecenchymal stem cells. Avicenna J Phytomed 2013; 3(2): 135-42.
[PMID: 25050267]

CHAPTER 6

Exploration of Dill Seeds (*Anethum Graveolens*): An Ayurpharmacomic Approach

Kounaina Khan[1], S Aishwarya[2], Pankaj Satapathy[2], Veena SM[3], Govindappa Melappa[4], Farhan Zameer[2,*], Shivaprasad Hudeda[1,*] and Sunil S. More[2,*]

[1] *Department of Dravyaguna, JSS Ayurvedic Medical College, Lalithadripura, Mysuru - 570 028, Karnataka, India*

[2] *School of Basic and Applied Sciences, Department of Biological Sciences, Dayananda Sagar University, Shavige Malleshwara Hills, Kumaraswamy Layout, Bengaluru - 560 078, Karnataka, India*

[3] *Department of Biotechnology, Sapthagiri Engineering College, Bangalore, India*

[4] *Department of Biotechnology, Dayananda Sagar College of Engineering, Dayananda Sagar Institutions, Shavige Malleshwara Hills, Kumaraswamy Layout, Bengaluru - 560 078, Karnataka, India*

Abstract: Since time immemorial, traditional medicine, largely Ayurveda, has established the usability and proficiency of many natural herbs and their formulations in curing ailments. However, the Asian continent or to be specific, India, could be considered as the "Land of Spices". The saga of food-spice-medicine recipes has been passed down to several generations with a motto to "Make Food as Medicine". One such exotic and the extensively used herb is *Anethum Graveolens* (Dill). This herb has the potential for various bioactivities. The whole plant, used as vrushya (a natural aphrodisiac), vataghna (balance vata) quenching excess free radicals, against vrana (non-healing wounds), shoola (abdominal colic pain), cure disorders and ulcers in eyes, plays a vital role in enema during panchakarma (bastikarma), functions as a galactagogue, inhibits uterine fibroids, increases milk secretion during lactation and above all enhances the taste of the food. With this background, a major lacuna is with an understanding of the functionality and mechanism of action at a molecular level. Hence, this chapter highlights the therapeutic potential of Dill seeds and their probable targets with modern knowledge and implications using ayurpharmacomic approach (understanding classical herbal formulation and exploring their pharmacological attributes with advanced -omic studies as tools). Further, virtual screening was performed to evaluate the structure-activity relationship (SAR) between lead phytobioactives and their pathological biomarkers/targets. These studies will enable a better understanding of potential pathways in developing newer therapeutic targets for future drug design and development, which would facilitate prime phytobioactive candidates to be subjected to clinical trials and drug approval.

* **Corresponding author Sunil S. More:** School of Basic and Applied Sciences, Department of Biological Sciences, Dayananda Sagar University, Shavige Malleshwara Hills, Kumaraswamy Layout, Bengaluru - 560 078, Karnataka, India; Tel: 0091-8073246552; E-mail drsunil@dsu.edu.in

Atta-ur-Rahman, M. Iqbal Choudhary & Sammer Yousuf

Keywords: Clinical studies, Dill seeds, Formulations, Phytobioactives, Pharmacology, Structure-activity relationship (SAR), Traditional medicine, Therapeutics.

INTRODUCTION

Anethum Graveolens L. is an annual herb that is commonly known as dill belonging to the Umbelliferae family growing in the Mediterranean region, Southern Asia and Europe. *Anethum Graveolens*/sowa is traditionally known as Shatapuspa, meaning a hundred flowers [1]. It is used as traditional ayurvedic medicine since ancient times to treat a variety of diseases. It is a plant that has a beautiful sweet fragrance; the genus is derived from the Greek word aneeson or aneeton, meaning a strong smell. Shatapushpa is one of the important drugs used in Ayurveda. Acharya Kashyapa has described its many other medicinal properties in a separate chapter called *"Shatapushpa Shatavari Kalpadhyaya"*. It grows up to 90cm tall in loose soil with yellow flowers and an aromatic odor. The leaves of the plant are arranged in an alternative manner on a slender stem and the fruits are oval, compressed, with dark lines, and a taste like caraway seeds [2]. Screening of phytochemicals (Fig. **1**) confirmed the presence of terpenoids, flavonoids, cardiac glycosides and tannins in the stem, root, and leaves. The most potent phytomolecules present in dill include carvone, limonene, α-phellandrene, β-phellandrene, myristicin, apiole, umbelliferone, anethole and P-anisaldehyde [3]. This herb inhibits the growth of carrots but is a good associate for lettuce, cabbages, onions, and corn. The yellow color of the flower attracts the bees, flies, and wasps for plant resources like nectar and pollens. When dill and coriander are planted together, they have the best pest controlling activity [4]. Dill serves as a host for parasitoid wasps such as *Cotesia glomerata, Pediobius foveolatus,* and *Edovum puttleri,* which parasitize caterpillars that feed on Dill, among other plant species [5]. Seventeen different volatile compounds have been identified in this plant from the seeds and inflorescence. Dill essential oil is found to have more therapeutic importance and is used to treat diseases; it is pale yellow with a fruity odor and acrid taste. Dill oil consists of d-carvone (23.1%), d-limonene (45%), eugenol, anethole, phenolic acids, α-phellandrene, coumarins, flavonoids, umbelliferones and triterpenes [6]. Dill essential oil is synthesized through the mevalonic acid pathway and shikimic acid pathway for terpenes and aromatic polypropanoids, respectively [7, 6].

There are various gynecological disorders seen in females by the impairment of the hypothalamic-pituitary-ovarian axis (HPO) due to the adoption of modern lifestyle, different dietary habits, physiological and psychological stress and sedentary lifestyle (Fig. **2**). In the Ayurvedic system of medicine, there are various herbs and formulations described for the prevention and management of gynecological problems in females, among which *Shatapushpa* has been described in ancient text. Importance was given by Kashyapa by describing properties like *Ritupravartini, Yonisukra vishodhini, Putraprd* and *Viryakari* hence it is used in *Anartava* (amenorrhoea), *Viphala Artava* (anovulatory cycles), *Atyartava* (menorrhagia), *Alpaartava* (hypomenorrhea), *Kashtartava* (dysmenorrhoea), *Rajonirvrutti* (menopause), *Yoni-shushkata* (dryness of vagina), *Vandhya & Shandhi* (infertility), *Rudhira Gulma* (useful in uterine fibroids) and *yonishoola* (pain in the vagina) [8]. This chapter describes the drug review, vernacular names in different languages, the biological, pharmacological, clinical and nutraceutical studies of the plant. This chapter also describes the structure of the potent phytomolecules and the structure-activity relationship of these molecules with various biomarkers that cause stress, inflammation, disorders, and diseases, which would be further explored as therapeutic targets for drug design and discovery.

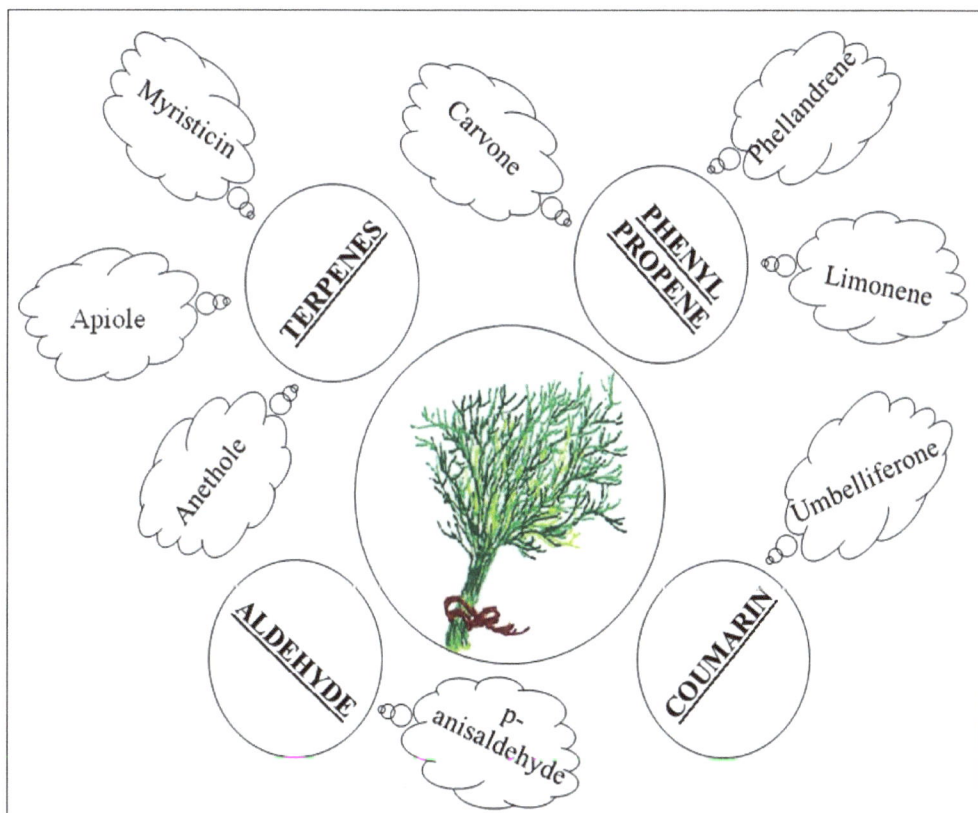

Fig. (1). Potent phytomolecules present in *Anethum Graveolens*.

DRUG REVIEW

BOTANICAL NAME: *Anethum sowa, Anethum Graveolens*

FAMILY: *Umbelliferae*

SANSKRITA: Sathapushpa, Chhatra, Shatahwa, Madhura, Mishi, Carvi

HINDI: Soyo

ENGLISH: Indian dill, dill, dill plant

TELUGU: Sadapa vittulu

TAMIL: Satakuppi

MARATHI: Shepur

KANNADA: Seed (Shataapu), Plant (Sabbasige soppu)

GUJRATHI: Suna

ARABIAN: Shibith

FARSI: Shebet, Sheneed

FRENCH: Aneth odorant

GERMAN: Dill

MORPHOLOGY

HABIT: An annual, glabrous aromatic herb growing up to 1 meter in height

LEAVES: Decompound with ultimate segments and filiform leaves 1.3 to 2.5 cm long

FLOWERS: Pale yellow in compound umbels form

FRUITS: Elliptical, dorsally compressed, 3.0 to 5.0 × 1.5 to 2.5 mm, glabrous, with three longitudinal ridges, narrowly winged, with two mericarps

FLOWERING: December to February

FRUITING: January to March [9, 6]

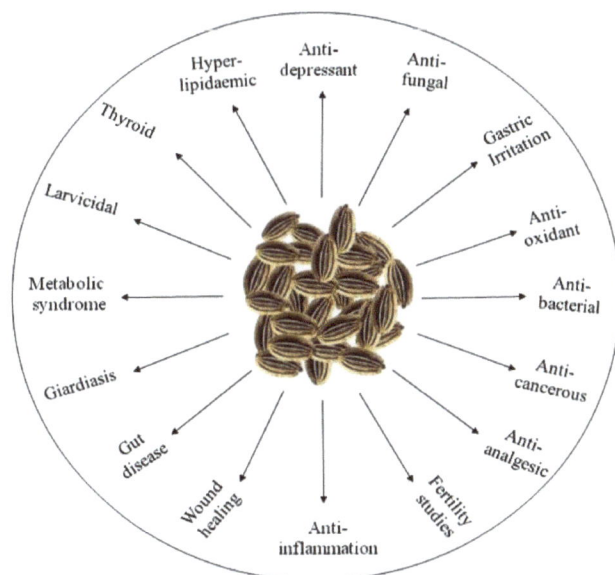

Fig. (2). Various diseases that are treated using Dill seeds.

BIOLOGICAL / PHARMACOLOGICAL / NUTRACEUTICAL ACTIVITIES OF SPICES AND CULINARY HERBS

Any deviation from the normal functioning of any organism, symptomatic or asymptomatic, leading to an abnormal state is a disease. Any organism in nature is susceptible to diseases, therefore, understanding the normal and the abnormal functioning of the organism is inevitable if we treat the disease. Dill seeds constitute phytobioactives that help in the treatment of several diseases (Fig. **2**); the major activities by the plant have been described comprehensively in this chapter. Further, Ayurpharmaco approach is the word coined in this chapter reflects the specific intent of exploring classical herbal ayurvedic formulations of dill seeds for their pharmacological and pharmaceutical attributes with –Omic tools like, proteomics and metabolomics for the better understanding of potential pathways and the mode of action of the phytobioactives which would lead into the development of newer drug/therapeutic targets. The data for structure-activity relationship (SAR) studies was exclusively generated for the chapter to provide a larger insight into the theme.

Metabolic Disorders

Metabolism is the process of breaking down food that contains carbohydrates, fats, and proteins to synthesize energy. Chemicals and enzymes in the body are involved in the breakdown of the food particles into sugars and acids to use it as the body's fuel. Metabolic disorders appear due to change in the process of metabolism by abnormal chemical reactions. Organs, including our liver, the pancreas can develop metabolic disorders where they become diseased and do not function normally. Lifestyle is also a major cause to acquire disorders [10]. It is prevalent in most of the places and it needs a high degree of attention. Most of the metabolic disorders have a synthetic cure, but natural medication is lacking. Dill acts as a natural alternative to treat metabolic disorders. Diabetes is a metabolic lifestyle disorder that is of two type's insulin-dependent type I diabetes and non-insulin dependent diabetes mellitus type II. Type I diabetes is an autoimmune disorder that is treated with exogenous insulin injection whereas type II diabetes that constitutes 90% of the cases can be managed by lifestyle changes [10]. Diabetes mellitus prevalence has risen in almost all parts of the world and has become the third most dangerous disease after cancer and cardiovascular diseases with high morbidity and mortality rate [11]. Defect in the pancreatic β-cells that function to produce insulin aggravates diabetic complications and free radicle production [12, 13]. Protein glycation further progresses complications related to diabetes, including nephropathy, neuropathy, and retinopathy [14]. Advanced glycation end products are formed in diabetic complications wherein detrimental stage free amino groups in the tissues or blood bind to excess glucose and disrupt the biomolecules, specifically proteins [15, 16]. Polyunsaturated fatty acids react with free radicals such as lipid peroxyl, peroxyl, hydrogen peroxide, superoxide anion and hydroxyl radicals leading to lipid peroxidation in diabetic condition [17, 18]. Antioxidant enzymes such as superoxide dismutase (SOD), catalase (CAT), glutathione S-transferase and glutathione peroxidase (GPx) inhibit the production of free radicals and eliminate the free radicals produced [19, 20]. There are multiple methods to treat and control diabetes through exercises, dietary control, hypoglycemic drugs and the administration of insulin [21, 22]. The administration of natural herbal plants enhanced the activities of these antioxidant enzymes in diabetes [23]. *Anethum Graveolens* essential oil reduced total cholesterol, low density, and very-low-density lipoproteins, whereas it enhanced high-density lipoprotein levels [6]. It is found that the flowers of the dill plant exhibited greater antioxidant activity due to the presence of flavonoids and phenolic proanthocyanidins than that of the leaf or seed extract [24]. *Anethum Graveolens* are found to bind to the bile acids present in the intestine and enhance the production of bile acids and fecal excretion inhibiting cholesterol absorption in the intestine causing anti-diabetic functions [6]. Phytomolecules such as carvone, α-phellandrene, and limonene at a concentration of 100 and 200 mg/kg is found to reduce cholesterol, fatty acid metabolism by reducing HMG-CoA reductase and acyl CoA carboxylase and also reduced fatty acid synthesis and improved lipoprotein metabolism [24, 25]. In a study to determine the antihyperglycemic effects of dill, leaves of the plant were collected and extracted with 80% ethanol. To determine the safe dosage of the plant extract twenty-eight rats were treated with different concentrations and it was found that 100 mg/kg was non-toxic and exhibited hypoglycemic effects. Wistar female rats were induced with hyperglycemia using corticosteroids and were treated with the plant extract. Dexamethasone enhanced lipid peroxidation and decreased the activities of antioxidant enzymes whereas the plant extract at a concentration of 100 mg/kg reversed the effect and also enhanced the thyroid hormonal level that was decreased proving the anti-diabetic effects of dill plant [26].

Thyroid

The thyroid gland is present in the frontal part of the neck below Adam's apple that produces thyroid hormones to regulate the metabolic rate. Thyroid disorder occurs when there is more or less production of thyroid hormones called hyperthyroidism and hypothyroidism respectively. Thyroid hormone synthesis takes place in the hypothalamus. Thyroid diseases are a major concern since 42 million people in India are suffering from thyroid disorders. It is a type of endocrine disease where a surgery called thyroidectomy is used as an alternative to reduce it [27]. Various treatments are being given to treat hyperthyroidism and hypothyroidism and the medication is well established [28].

A study was conducted to decipher the effect of dill on diabetes mellitus, T3, T4, and Thyroid-stimulating hormone (TSH) concentrations by Idiz *et al.* [29]. Female Wistar Albino rats were used as a model organism to induce and treat the condition. Leaves and stem of the plant were collected and extracted in ethanol at room temperature. Before treating the rats with the extract blood was drawn and the T3, T4 and TSH levels were assessed. Leaves and stem extracts were administered to the rats at different concentrations that included 50, 150 and 300 mg/ kg/ day. After the treatment with the extract for 30 days, then 300 mg/kg dose of the extract exhibited a high degree of decrease in the TSH level but there was no change observed in the T3 and T4 levels. This study suggests that dill extract can be used as a therapeutic agent to treat hyperthyroidism at a higher dosage [29].

Metabolic Syndrome

Metabolic syndrome is a cluster of metabolic disorders closely associated with stroke risk [30]. Within three months of stroke, survivors are prone to developing cognitive impairment. Cognitive impairment is a condition when a person has a disorder remembering, concentrating, making decisions and learning new things [31]. According to traditional folklore, food not only serves as energy and nutrition but also promotes health. Polyphenols present in food act as neuroprotectants. Polyphenols and diet that contains a high amount of anthocyanin are found to improve brain damage in an animal model induced with metabolic syndrome [32]. *Anethum Graveolens* and *Oryza sativa* are found to have neuroprotective [33], antioxidant [34] and anti-inflammatory activity [35].

A study was conducted combining dill and black stick rice creating OA extract, the extract contained phenolic compounds and flavonoids. The content in *O. sativa* and *A. graveolens* was much lower when compared to the combined extract. The major scavenger enzymes responsible for oxidative stress and neuron densities were lowered at a concentration of 50 mg/kg that included catalase (CAT), superoxide dismutase (SOD) and glutathione peroxidase (GSH-Px). In conclusion, brain damage and inflammation in the neurons and oxidative stress can be attenuated with the help of anthocyanins which were present in higher amounts in OA extract [36].

Accumulation of Lipid in Liver

Liver a vital organ responsible for numerous physiological processes in our body including immune system support, lipid and cholesterol balance, macronutrient metabolism, blood volume regulation, breakdown of xenobiotic compounds and endocrine control of growth signaling pathways [37]. In the last few decades, the main cause of death of people is due to heart diseases and alcoholic and non-alcoholic fatty liver disease [38]. People suffering from these conditions will have changes in low-density lipoprotein (LDL) and have a reduced amount of high-density lipoprotein cholesterol (HDL-C). In a study, male Syrian hamsters were induced with a high cholesterol diet for a month and sacrificed. Blood samples and the liver tissue were collected and the total cholesterol, biochemical factors, and triglyceride levels were determined. Dill tablets were prepared from the ethanolic extract of the seeds and filtered through Whatman 2 filter paper. Lactate dehydrogenase, alkaline phosphatase, aspartate transaminase, alanine transaminase, γ-glutamyl transferase, total bilirubin, direct bilirubin, triglyceride, total cholesterol, total antioxidant and malondialdehyde levels in hypercholesterolemic hamsters were normalized on treatment with these tablets at a concentration of 100 mg/kg and 300 mg/kg. Total protein and albumin concentrations were significantly increased in dill treated groups. These results deduce that dill not only reduces liver damage but also acts as an antioxidant [39].

Inflammation

When a pathogen or anything harmful affects our body, inflammation occurs which is a defensive mechanism adopted by the body against the pathogen. Inflammation is beneficial but prolonged or chronic inflammation leads to deadly diseases like cancer and rheumatoid arthritis [40]. Several synthetic drugs are available to treat chronic inflammation but they have been found to induce adverse side effects. Therefore to overcome the side effects caused by these drugs naturally available plant extracts are used to treat inflammatory diseases [41]. Dill leaves and seeds exhibit therapeutic potential such as antibacterial [42], antioxidant [43], appetizer [44], anti-bloating [45] and anti-spasmodic [46] activities. A study conducted by Mohensen *et al.* proved that the aqueous extract of the plant in sesame oil at a concentration of 100 mg tested on *Rattus rattus* induced with paw inflammation exhibited anti-inflammatory and analgesic effects [47].

Nitric oxide functions to regulate pathological, physiological and inflammatory responses [48, 49] overproduction of nitric oxide may lead to diseases such as tissue injuries, rheumatoid arthritis, atherosclerosis, septic shock and malignancy [48, 50]. In this study, *Anethum Graveolens* flower extract was used to treat lipopolysaccharide (LPS) induced inflammation in macrophage RAW 264.7 cell line. Lipopolysaccharide enhanced nitric oxide production, inhibited iNOS gene expression, increased COX-2, IL-1β gene expression, and IL-6 levels. LPS is found to activate P13K/Akt signaling pathway in-turn NF-kβ by the destruction of IkB [48, 51]. *Anethum Graveolens* flower extract treatment blocked ERK1/2, Akt, MAPK and p38 phosphorylation it also suppressed IkB degradation and inhibited nuclear translocation of NF-kβ at a concentration of 50 and 100 μg/mL. In conclusion, it was proved that the flower extract of dill has potent anti-inflammatory activity through regulation of iNOS expression through P13K/Akt and MAPK pathways [52].

Anti-Oxidant

Lately, the use of herbs, shrubs have allured abundant attention as an alternative therapy for inflammation for their lower toxicity and cost-effectiveness [53]. Moderate level or low level of reactive oxygen species (ROS) and reactive nitrogen species (RNS) are biologically important since they function as regulatory and signaling molecules [54]. High levels of ROS and RNS lead to oxidative stress leading to damage of all the types of biomolecules such as proteins, enzymes, lipids, carbohydrates, DNA and amino acids [55]. In normal condition, there is a proper balance between antioxidants and oxidants, any kind of disturbance to this equilibrium lead to oxidative stress. The accumulation of oxidative stress leads to chronic and degenerative disorders such as cancer, diabetes and Alzheimer's disease [56]. To treat such complexes the use of naturally available medicinal plants would be an effective method. Dill or sowa is a traditionally available plant that has several therapeutic properties. Therefore to evaluate the anti-oxidant effects of dill, different extracts using petroleum ether, n-butanol, ethyl acetate, and water fractions were prepared. To examine the cytotoxicity LPS-induced macrophages RAW264.7 isolated from mice were treated with the extracts and it was found that extracts below the concentration of 100 µg/mL were non-toxic. Nitric oxide synthase (iNOS) decreased on treatment with the extracts and slight changes were observed in the levels of interleukins 1 and 6. Among all the fractions ethyl acetate and petroleum ether fractions exhibited the best antioxidant and anti-inflammatory activity [57].

Antidepressant and Analgesic Activity

Depression is a mood disorder that may be caused due to the following reasons: (i) family history, (ii) childhood trauma, (iii) brain structure, (iv) drug use, (v) low self-esteem, (vi) personal history of mental illness (v) medical conditions like insomnia, chronic pain, chronic illness and due to attention deficit hyperactivity disorder [58]. *A. graveolens* achenes powder was extracted in aqueous decoction where tannins and flavonoids were found in higher amounts. The plantar test was conducted to determine the analgesic effect of the extract against the standard tramadol the result showed that the extract prolonged the time of pain tolerance. The concentration of 250 mg/kg and 100mg/kg exhibited a marked reduction in the depression level and nociceptive effect [59].

Gut Disease

Cannabis sativa is the oldest available domesticated traditional plant that is made up of 90% of fatty acid and high levels of vitamins, β-carotene, and minerals [60]. Dill seeds are rich in dill apiole [61], carvone and limonene [62]. The gut is known as the second brain changes in the gut may lead to disturbance in metabolism. To understand gut health, broiler chicken were treated with hemp and dill seeds diet and examined. There were no changes observed in the weight of the birds. Serum enzymes such as amino transaminase (AST) and alanine aminotransaminase (ALT) concentrations were lowered preventing hepatic damage. In the jejunum and caecum, there is a lowered amount of coliforms observed whereas lactobacilli species had proliferated in both portions of the intestine. Hemp and dill seeds at a concentration of 0.2% and 0.3% respectively, exhibited the best enzyme profile and gut health [63].

Gastric Irritation

Lesions in the stomach cause gastritis and ulcers causing an increase in the pH of the stomach acid [64]. Extracts of dill seeds have found to have effective anti-ulcer and anti-secretary activity in male albino BALB/c mice. Flavonoids isolated from the extract isorhamnetin 3-O-beta-D-glucuronide and quercetin 3-O-beta-D-glucuronide have been found to exhibit these activities [65]. Mice were induced to have gastric lesions with the help of HCl and were used to examine the effect of the extract. Oral administration of the aqueous extract at a concentration of 0.17

g/kg and 0.07 g/kg of ethanolic extracts and intraperitoneal application of the aqueous and ethanolic extract at a concentration of 0.02g/kg and 0.03 g/kg, respectively, exhibited best anti-ulcer and anti-secretary activity [66].

Microbial Diseases

Microbes are minute microscopic single-celled organisms that can cause diseases in humans also called pathogens. Whereas some class of bacteria such as actinomycetes can produce antibiotics such as nocardicin and streptomycin [67]. Bacteria present in the gut function to the breakdown of ingested food and help in absorption protecting the body. The flora present in the gut defines the person, every possible mechanism in the body is found to be regulated by these microorganisms present in the gut. Some pathogens that cause diseases in humans include *Salmonella typhi, Klebsiella pneumoniae, Shigella flexneri,* and *Staphylococcus aureus* [67].

Bacterial Diseases

Microbial strains have developed resistance to multiple drugs due to the surplus use of antibiotics against infectious diseases. Therefore the use of natural herbal medicine to treat various infections has garnered interest [68]. Gurinder *et al* conducted a study to test the anti-bacterial effect of three plants belonging to the family Umbelliferae namely, *Anethum Graveolens* L., *Trachyspermum ammi* L., and *Foeniculum vulgare* Mill. These plants are used to treat gastrointestinal disorders, used as spices, condiments, and essential oils have known to possess diuretic properties [69]. Aqueous and organic extracts of the seeds were prepared and their anti-bacterial properties were tested through the agar diffusion method. Hot water extract of all the three seeds exhibited better zone of inhibition at a concentration of 200 mg/mL compared to all other extracts within 10 hours and there was no re-growth observed. 90-92% of *Staphylococcus aureus* was inhibited by the seeds extract. In conclusion, the seeds of these plants could be used as a therapeutic anti-bacterial agent [70].

Bacterial cells communicate to regulate the expression of genes involved in biofilm formation, enzyme secretion, production of pigment and bacterial motility by a process known as quorum sensing [71]. *Serratia marcescens* is a pathogenic bacterium responsible for urinary tract infection resistant to antibiotics involved in causing hazardous infections. In the hunt of quorum sensing inhibitory (QSI) compounds, phytochemicals have been examined because of their non-toxic nature [72]. To investigate antibiofilm and antipathogenic activities, dill plant was selected since it is extensively used as spices, condiments, to treat gastrointestinal disorders, mental disorders and urinary complaints [73]. Methanolic extract of the plant was tested using biosensor strains *Chromobacterium violaceum CV026* and

Chromobacterium violaceum ATCC 1247. On treatment with the extract, genes *bsmA, flhD* and *fimC* were down-regulated compared to the control. Therefore the biofilm formation in the early stages itself was inhibited due to reduced motility of the bacteria. The quorum-sensing mechanism was inhibited by 3-O-methyl ellagic acid present in the methanolic extract of the plant concluding that the seeds have an anti-quorum sensing mechanism [74].

Fungal Diseases

Fungal diseases are a major concern these days since the diagnosis is very difficult due to non-specific symptoms. Fungi is difficult to be grown under *in-vitro* culture conditions antibodies may cross-react, histopathological diagnosis is formidable, therefore diagnosis and treatment are lacking with fungal diseases [75]. *Candida* species cause serious fungal infections that cause candidiasis where *C. albicans* are the most predominant virulent species that are present in infected bloodstreams, on oral mucosal layers and in vaginal infections [76]. Yuxin *et al.* made use of dill essential oil to determine the anti-fungal effect against *C. albicans* ATCC 64550 strain. Apoptosis of yeast was due to chromatin condensation and DNA fragmentation. Dill essential oil was found to cause serious damage to the strain by causing nuclear fragmentation, chromatin condensation through ROS accumulation [77]. Essential oil promotes the production of cytochrome C in-turn triggering the release of Apaf-1 and procaspase-9 which form an apoptosome. This apoptosome functions to activate caspase-9 and enforces the metacaspase cascade to induce apoptosis through a metacaspase-dependent apoptotic pathway in *C. albicans* ATCC 64550 [78].

Larvicidal Effects

Malaria caused by *Anopheles stephensi* is found to be the major vector that has brought about 429,000 deaths and 212 million cases around the world [79]. An increase in modernization and lack of sanitation has led to an increase in the population of mosquitoes. These mosquitoes have grown resistance to chemical larvicides on the continuous application due to environmental pollution [80]. Essential oils obtained from plants are used as larvicides in industries rather than the chemically available ones [81]. Mahmoud *et al.* conducted a study to determine the effect of dill essential oil against third and fourth instar larvae of *An. stephensi.* By the process of spontaneous emulsification, nanoemulsions of the essential oil were prepared. In the essential oil high amounts of carvone, dill ether, p-cymenealpha, cis-sabinol, and alpha-phellandrene were preset. The nanoemulsions with a particle size distribution of less than two exhibited the best larvicidal activity against *A. stephensi* [82].

Fertility Studies

Fertility is the ability to undergo nine months of gestation period to give birth to a child. Fertility plays a major role in population control and growth; many steroidal remedies are taken as anti-fertility agents which in the long run has innumerable side effects. Therefore there is a need for herbal remedy as anti-fertility agents. An oral contraceptive that is used to control fertility taken for a prolonged period leads to irregularities in the menstrual cycle and causes breast cancer. Men are less exposed to such contraceptives because of the limited availability of such tablets for men in birth control [83]. Monsefi *et al.* used Wistar rats to determine the anti-fertility effect of the ethanolic extract of dill seeds. Extract administered at a concentration of 0.45 g/kg exhibited the best anti-fertility activity [84]. The antifertility effect of various solvent extracts of Dill seeds was also tested in female rats. The solvents that were used for extraction included aqueous, n-butanol, chloroform and ether. The aqueous and n-butanol extracts exhibited an anti-fertility effect on the rats which could not conceive. This effect was confirmed through mating experiments by fetching a vaginal smear of the female rats that had mated and there was no pregnancy observed [85].

Apart from this, another experiment was conducted on ovarian granulosa cells and immature oocytes which were collected from immature superovulated Balb/c female mice. Aqueous extract of dill seeds was tested for its anti-fertility effect at a concentration of 1000 μg/mL and it was found to be non-toxic however the viability of these cells reduced subsequently at a concentration of 10000 μg/mL. The high concentration of Dill aqueous extract led to the increase in the levels of lipid droplets, estrogen, progesterone, and alkaline phosphatase. The result of dill seeds on oocytes confirmed its anti-fertility effects [86].

Other Activities

Wound Healing

Wound healing is an intricate method that comprises of interdependent stages such as proliferation, remodeling, inflammation, and homeostasis [87]. Apoptosis plays a major role in regulating inflammatory response and to activate the process of normal wound healing [88]. Molecules including Bcl-2, caspase-3, Bcl-XL, and p53 are known to be involved in the wound healing process. Increased expression of p53 enhances the apoptosis of the inflammatory cells and their eradication however Bcl-2 inhibits apoptosis and enhances cellular proliferation [89]. The major organisms that are present in the infected wounds include methicillin-resistant *Staphylococcus aureus* and *Pseudomonas aeruginosa*. Naturally available plant essential oils can inhibit the growth of the bacteria and enhances the wound healing process [90]. Dill essential oil (DEO) was used to test its anti-microbial property in BALB/c male mice using primary rabbit anti-mouse monoclonal antibodies for p53 and Bcl-2. DEO enhances the expression of p53, caspase-3, and Bcl-2 where they induce apoptosis and promote cellular proliferation respectively [91]. This study concluded that DEO reduced the inflammatory stages by inducing apoptosis and up-regulating p53 and caspase-3. Dill essential consists of major compounds such as carvone, α-phellandrene, and p-cymene that are involved in wound healing. It is found to enhance angiogenesis through the activation of fibroblast growth factor-2 and vascular endothelial growth factor that enhances the deposition and biosynthesis of collagen confirming its use in ointments would intensify the process of wound healing [92].

Cancer

Cancer is the second most leading cause of mortality; 9.6 million people around the world are dying of cancer and its types according to the World Health Organization [93]. The major types of cancer include sarcoma, carcinoma, lymphoma, leukemia, and melanoma. Hepatocellular carcinoma (HCC) is the fifth universal cancer with the second-highest mortality rate compared to all other cancers [94]. The available treatments for hepatocellular carcinoma include tumor embolization, tumor ablation, radiation therapy and chemotherapy [95] however these therapies are costly and have various side effects [96]. Herbal plant-based medicines have been found to contain anti-cancer compounds that can fight against cancers [96]. *Anethum Graveolens* L. is a culinary herb that has been extensively used in ethnopharmacological traditional medicine to treat various diseases including cancer, it is found to be effective in uterus cancer [97]. Therefore ethyl acetate fraction of dill seed were used to determine its effect on hepatocellular carcinoma cell line (HepG2) and normal human fibroblast cell line (HDFa). HepG2 cells underwent apoptosis on treatment with the extract at a concentration of 0.6 and 0.8 mg/mL through various mechanisms including cell shrinkage, nuclear condensation, membrane disruption and blebbing. Ethyl acetate fraction activates caspase 8 and caspase 9, that in-turn activates the intrinsic mitochondrial pathway to induce apoptosis of the HepG2 cells through caspase 3 [98].

CLINICAL STUDIES ON SPICES AND CULINARY HERBS-BASED FORMULATIONS AND ITS CONSTITUENTS

Giardiasis

Giardia lamblia is a flagellated intestinal protozoan that causes giardiasis characterized by weight loss, malabsorption, diarrhea, bloating and abdominal cramps [99]. Giardiasis occurs through the consumption of water or food that is contaminated with infected feces or person-to-person transmission [100]. Chemotherapy and metronidazole (Met) is the existing treatment for giardiasis however Met-resistant strains of the pathogen and the parasite are further reasons for alternate therapy [101]. Dill is employed to determine its effect in pediatric patients suffering from the disease. Aqueous extract of the seeds was prepared and administered at a concentration of 1mL 3 times a day for 5 days. After 5 days the stool samples did not contain any parasite and were completely reduced whereas patients treated with Met for 5 days reduced the incidence of the parasite proving that dill is a potent anti-giardia culinary herb [102].

Labour Pain

Delivery is a physiological mechanism that commences with pain causing anxiety, fatigue and negative effects on labor progress [103]. Excessive pain leads to the release of cortisol and catecholamine that further enhances the pain and prolongs labor. In this scenario, it will lead to fatal complications including improper oxygen supply, head compression, perineal trauma and fetal death [104]. *Anethum Graveolens* has been used as a traditional herbal medicine because of its therapeutic properties. To authenticate the effect of dill seeds on pain intensity during labor stages, clinical trials were carried out on women. Dill seeds (10g) were boiled in 100 cc water and administered to the patients. The results were as follows: the duration of the labor stages was lower, better contractions of the uterus, increased dilation and better progress of delivery concluding that dill seeds can decrease pain intensity during labor stages [105].

DILL SEEDS – AN AYURVEDIC PERSPECTIVE AND THEIR FORMULATIONS

External Applications

According to Acharya Charaka in Shushka, Arsha/hemorrhoids should be fomented with lumps of Vacha and Shatapushpa mixed with unctuous substances [106]. In Vata predominant Vata Rakta (Gout) Paste of Atasi (linseed), Eranda (castor seeds) and Shatapushpa seeds pounded with milk, is used for local application to remove Shoola (pain) (Charaka samhita Vatarakta chikitsa) [107]. Vishahara lepa: Paste of Shatpushpa mixed with rock salt and Ghee has been used for local application to counteract Bees poison (Bhela Samhita Visha/216).

Internal Usage

Bastikarma (enema): It is widely used as a kalka in basti therapy, it helps to regularize the apana vata. It is also used in treating Agnimandhya (dyspepsia), Aruchi (anorexia) and Vamana (emesis) - because of its Usna, Tikshna, Pittakrit,

Deepana, Pachana, Ruchidayaka, Vatanulomana properties (Table **1**). Rasayana: According to Acharya Kashyapa, Shatapushpa promotes intellect within a month when it is given with honey and Ghee (Table **2**) [108].

Table 1. Rasa panchaka/properties.

Rasa (taste)	Madhura (sweet), Katu (pungent), Tikta (Bitter)
Guna (qualities)	Laghu (easy to digest), Teekshna (piercing/ enters the deeper tissues), Ruksha (dry)
Virya (potency)	Ushna (hot)
Vipaka (conversion in taste after digestion)	Katu (pungent)
Effect on Doshas	Pitta vardhaka (increases Pitta, balances Kapha and Vata)

Table 2. Classical categorization.

According to Charaka Samhita	Asthapanopaga mahakashaya (used in decoction enema preparation) Anuvasanopaga mahakashaya (used in oil enema preparations)
Acoording to Sushruta Samhita	Asthapana gana
According to Kashyapa Samhita	Shatapushpa Shatavari kalpa Rasayana (tonic/rejuvenative)
Dhanvantari Nighuntu	Shatapushpadi varga
Bhavaprakasha Nighuntu	Haritakyadi varga
Kaiyadeva Nighuntu	Aushadha varga
Raj Nighuntu	Shatahwadi varga

According to Acharya Kashyapa, it is used in different conditions with different Anupanas (vehicle) [109].

For:

Bala Vardhan - Taila

Pleeha roga - Katu taila

Agnivriddhi - Madhu

Rupa Vardhan - Ksheer & Sarpi

Kamala, Pandu and Shotha - Mahisha ksheer and Mutra

Kushta - Khadiravari

Gulma - Eranda taila

Pharmacological Uuses of Shatapushpa in Different Gynecological Disorders with Its Probable Mode of Action

Anulomana Karma of shatapushpa will cause "Doshanam Samshosana" and facilitate the free movement of Apana Vayu. As Apana vayu helps in the production of artava hence it acts as Rajah pravartaka (emmenagogue) (Table **3**) [110] and it relieves Dysmenorrhea (kashtartava) due to inhibition of prostaglandin production and antispasmodic action [111, 112].

Table 3. Probable mode of action.

Dosha Karma	Dhatu Karma	Mala Karma	Sroto Karma
Vatakaphashamaka			
Madhura rasa & Ushna virya- vata↓ Katu & tikta rasa, Katu vipaka and ushna virya- kapha↓	rasavardhaka/raktavardhaka	Anulomana	Srotoshodhaka: Katu rasa and Ruksha, Tikshna Guna, remove obstruction in channels by Lekhana karma, Kapha Vilayan helps in srotoshodhana

Phytoestrogens exert their effect in selective estrogen receptor modulators (SERM). Through this SERM action, they inhibit the enzymatic conversion of endogenous oestrone to oestradiol and also possess intrinsic estrogen activity useful in reducing the menopausal effects (like hot flush, vaginitis, anxiety, and osteoporosis).

Anartava and Atyartava: Shatapushpa contains monoterpenes such as carvone, limonene, and trans-anethole and some flavonoids such as kaempferol and vicenin. Kaempferol, trans-anethole and limonene exhibit phytoestrogenic activity. Phytoestrogen can be useful in both hyper estrogenic and hypoestrogenic state in the body due to their adaptogenic activity. Thus depending on the target tissue, it may be estrogenic and anti-estrogenic therefore it is useful in Anartava (amenorrhoea), Viphala Artava, (anovulation) and Atyartava (menorrhagia).

Pelvic inflammatory disease (PID): through its anti-inflammatory and antibacterial actions it can also be used in vaginal infections [113]. (*A. graveolens* showed a broad-spectrum of antibacterial activity against *S. aureus, E. coli, P. aeruginosa, S. typhimurium, Shigella flexneri,* and *Salmonella typhii*) to cure the PID.

Yoni Shushkata (dryness of vagina): shatapushpa taila pichu (tampon) is used.

PHYTOCHEMISTRY OF SPICES AND CULINARY HERBS

Widely used phytomolecules in *Anethum Graveolens* including carvone, limonene, and umbelliferone are known for their therapeutic activities can also be isolated from different plants. Carvone is a monoterpene ketone that can be isolated from *Mentha spicata* (spearmint) essential oil and any plant belonging to the family *Lamiaceae* and also from *Lippia alba* commonly known as bushy mat grass [114]. Limonene is a cyclic monoterpene aliphatic hydrocarbon that is mainly present in citrus fruits [115]. Umbelliferone is a phenylpropanoid that is present in the plants belonging to *Umbelliferae* family such as coriander, carrot, and banana [116]. Carvone, limonene, and umbelliferone are molecules known to possess anti-microbial, anti-diabetic, analgesic, anti-depressant, anti-cancer, and leishmanicidal activities. Previous studies have been executed from our lab where phytochemicals such as umbelliferone and lupeol [117] and phytosterols such as stigmasterol and sitosterol [118] have been isolated, purified and characterized from *Musa* sp. var. Nanjangud Rasa Bale. Furthermore, these isolated phytomolecules were tested for its anti-diabetic activity in Wistar rats induced with diabetes with the help of alloxan. Umbelliferone and lupeol were isolated from the inflorescence whereas stigmasterol and β-sitosterol were isolated from the pseudostem of the plant. Administration of the ethanolic extract of stigmasterol and β-sitosterol and umbelliferone and lupeol enhanced the production of insulin by restoring β-cells and also positively regulated glycogen storage pathways and glucose utilization. These molecules are found to possess anti-diabetic, anti-oxidant [119], anti-hyperglycemic properties [120].

In all the studies that have been performed, *in silico* studies of the phytomolecules present in *Anethum Graveolens* has not been executed, to provide a new touchstone to the paper, structure and activity relationship studies have been carried out and incorporated. The top phytomolecules and their activity have been represented below correspondingly. These studies give an insight into the potent phytomolecules that is present in different parts of the plants and their bioactivities (Fig. 3). The efficient targets of different disorders or diseases have been selected for the study. The result gives us a corollary to perform the wet lab experiments and to prove the results (Table 4).

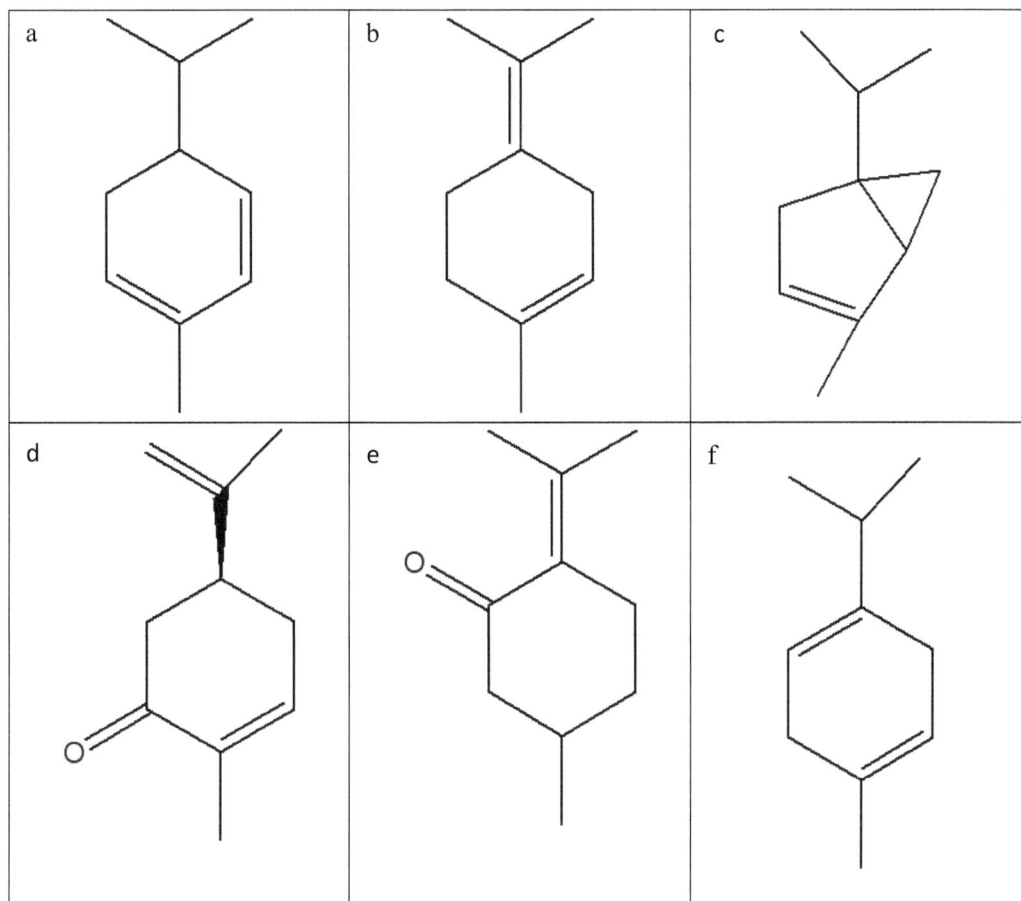

Fig. 3 contd.....

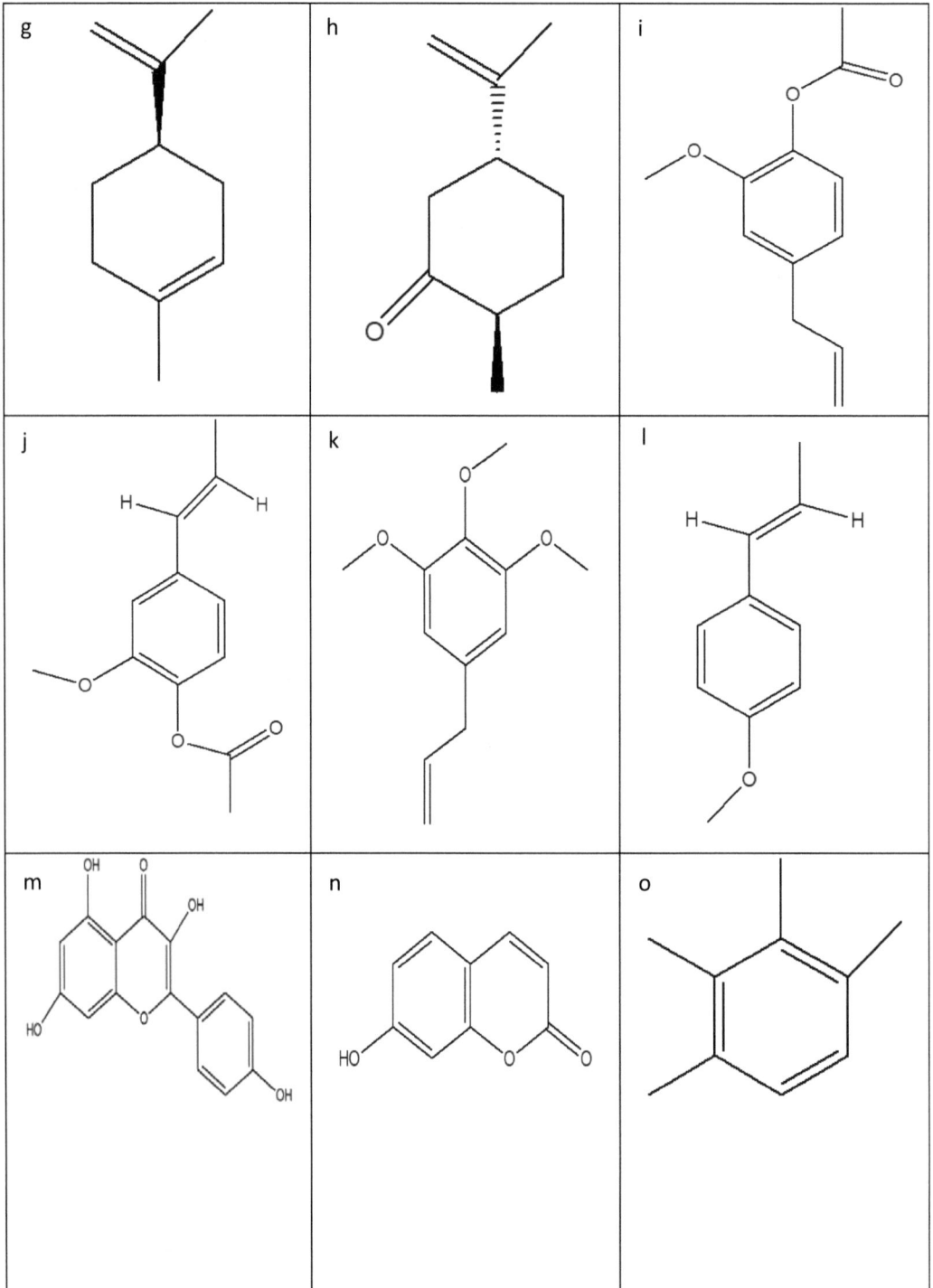

Fig. 3 contd.....

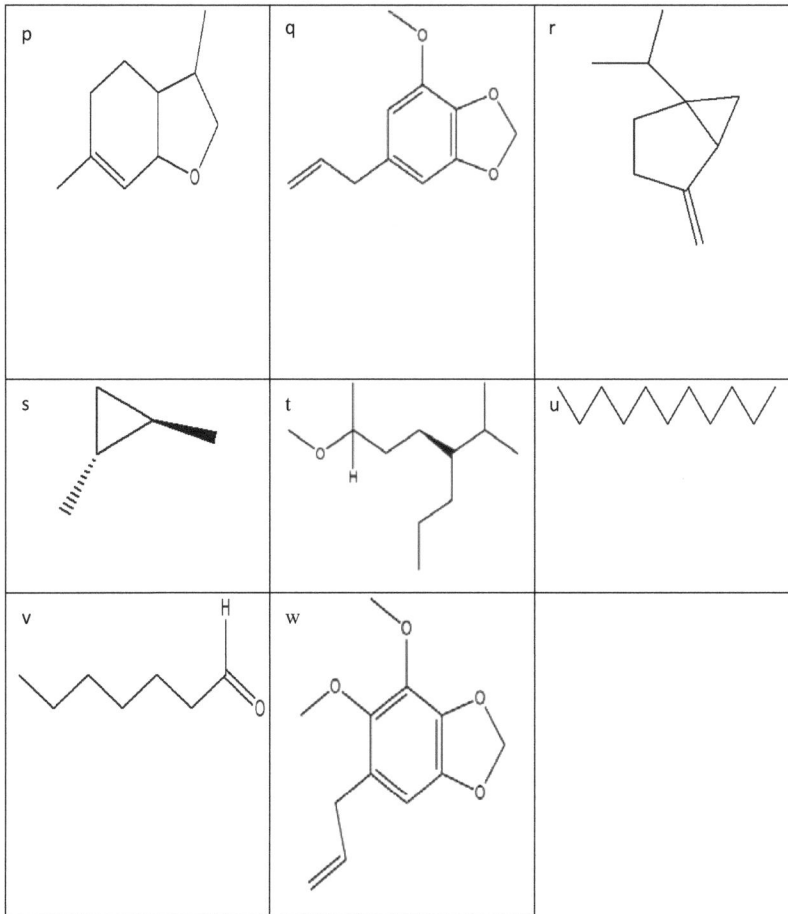

Fig. (3). (a) α- Phellandrene, (b) α-terpinolene, (c) α-thujene, (d) d-carvone, (e) pulegone, (f) γ-terpinene, (g) d-limonene, (h) d-dihydrocarvone, (i) eugenol acetate, (j) isoeugenol acetate, (k) elemicin, (l) trans-anethole, (m) kaempferol, (n) umbelliferone, (o) prehnitene, (p) dill ether, (q) myristicin, (r) sabinene, (s) trans-1,2-dimethylcyclopropane, (t) cis-limonene oxide, (u) undecane (v) heptanal, (w) dillapiole.

Table 4. Diseases that are treated with dill seeds and their dosage and model organisms used.

Disease	Model	Extract Used	Dose	Markers	Reference
Thyroid	Female Wistar albino rats	Ethanolic	300 mg/kg	T3,T4,TSH	[29]
Metabolic syndrome condition	Male Wistar rats	Ethanolic	--	MDA, SOD and GSH-px, AcHE, IL-6, and TNF-α	[36]

(Table 4) cont.....

Disease	Model	Extract Used	Dose	Markers	Reference
Hepato-protective	Male wistar rats	Tablets	100 mg/kg & 300 mg/kg	Liver cholesterol, triglyceride, malondialdehyde (MDA), total antioxidant capacity (TAC) and catalase (CAT)	[56]
Anti-depressant and Analgesic	Wistar rats	Aqueous	250 mg/kg & 1 g/kg	Nociseption	[59]
Hyper-cholesterolemia	Golden Syrian male hamsters	Hydro-alcoholic	200 mg/kg	HMG-CoA reductase	[39]
Gut health	Broiler Chicken	Seeds	0.3%	Amino transaminase and Alaniamino transaminase	[63]
Anti-ulcer	Male albino mice BALB/c	Aqueous and Ethanolic	0.17 g/kg & 0.07 g/kg	Gastric lesions	[41]
Inflammation	Rat	Oil	100 mg/kg	Behavioural	[47]
	RAW264.7cell line	Ethanolic	25-100 µg/mL	iNOS, IL1& IL6	[57]
Larvicidal	*Anopheles stephensi*	Oil	1.20%	--	[82]
Quorum sensing	*S. marcescens*	Methanolic	256 µg/mL	Gene expression	[74]
Anti-fungal	*Candida albicans*	Oil	--	Cyt C	[77]
Fertility	Male wistar rats	Ethanolic	0.045 g/kg & 0.45 g/kg	--	[84]
	Female rats	Aqueous and N-butanol	0.045 g/kg & 0.45 g/kg	Estradiol	[85]
	Granular cells and oocytes		10000 µg/ml	Estrogen, progesterone & alkaline phosphatase	[86]
Wound healing	BALB/c Mice	oil	--	Bcl-2, P53, caspase-3, VEGF, FGF-2	[91]
Cancer	HepG2 cell	Ethyl acetate	0.5 & 0.6 mg/ml	--	[98]

(Table 4) cont.....

Disease	Model	Extract Used	Dose	Markers	Reference
Repellant	German cockroaches	oil	2.5 $\mu g/cm^2$	--	[121]
Labour	Clinical	Raw	10 g	--	[105]
Giardiasis	Clinical	Aqueous	1ml	--	[122]

STRUCTURE-ACTIVITY RELATIONSHIP (SAR) STUDIES

Molecular docking studies were executed to establish a correlation between the top three potent phytomolecules (carvone, limonene, and umbelliferone) present in dill seeds. Any disorder has three major common pathways stress leading to inflammation and finally a disease, therefore our main focus on cancer. Therefore all the three pathways were chosen and the targets were screened and SAR studies were performed. Stress-related targets catalase and superoxide dismutase were employed for the study with accession number in RCSB Protein Data Bank (PDB, https://www.rcsb.org/): 1DGB and 2ADQ, respectively. Inflammatory targets such as cyclooxygenase-2 and lipooxygenase with accession number 1CX2 and 1YGE were chosen respectively. Cancer targets like p53-Mdm2 and epidermal growth factor receptor with accession number 4HFZ and 2GS2 were preferred for the study, respectively. The potent phytomolecules (ligands) were docked into the active site using Molecular docking software PATCH Dock with default parameters. PATCH Dock is an algorithm that is used to calculate the docking modes of small molecules into the active sites based on the shape complementarity. Molecular docking of the molecules revealed the atomic contact energy (ACE) and the amino acid binding residues that are as depicted in Tables **5**, **6** and **7**. The structures of the ligands were constructed using Dundee PRODRG server [123] which reduces the energy and standardizes the conformation of the side chains. The precise location of the binding site and the potentiality of the ligand to bind to the active site were determined using an automated docking software, molegro virtual docker 2008, version 3.2.1 (Molegro ApS, Aarhus, Denmark, http://molegro.com), that is based on guided differential evolution and a force filed based screening function [124]. With the help of Clustering methods, the possible binding conformations and orientations were determined. The enzyme was visualized using the sequence option. The binding site was calculated within a spacing range so that the binding site was well sampled with a grid resolution of 0.3 Å. Using MolDock optimizer algorithm the ligand was docked into the grid and the interactions were analyzed using detailed energy estimates. The software was utilized to identify hydrogen bonds and hydrophobic interactions between residues at the active site and the ligand.

Table 5. Docking sites and their atomic contact energy values for stress disorder.

Name of the Biomarker	Name of the Compound	Details of H-bond interaction No. of bonds	Atomic contact Energy (ACE) Values	Amino acid residues on docked domains
Catalase (1DGB)	Carvone	0	-97.22	Val 74, His 75, Ser 114, Arg 112
	Limonene	0	-144.54	Met 339
	Umbelliferone	0	-69.79	Arg 72, Phe 334, His 362
	Donazepril	4	-250.63	Gly 121, Ser 122, Ser 254, Pro 258, Ala 117, Gly 121, Ser 122, Ala 117, Gly121, Ser 122, Ala 123, Arg 127, Lys 177, Ser 254, Gln 255, Pro 258
SOD (superoxide dismutase) (2ADQ)	Carvone	0	-143.67	Gly 179, Ile 223, Thr 250, Ala 254, Ser 255
	Limonene	0	-130.73	Ile 223, Ala 254
	Umbelliferone	3	-147.66	Thr 202, Asp 203, Ile 223, Ser 255
	Donazepril	5	-365.13	Val 159, Gly 251, Val 272, Gly 272, Leu 274, Gly 275, Ser 276, Thr 279, Val 296, Phe 297, Arg 298

Table 6. Docking sites and their atomic contact energy values for inflammation.

Name of the Biomarker	Name of the Compound	Details of H-bond interaction No. of bond	Atomic contact Energy (ACE) Values	Amino acid residues on docked domains
COX2 (Cyclooxygenase-2) (1CX2)	Carvone	0	-157.74	-
	Limonene	0	-148.22	Leu 352, tyr 355, Tyr 385, Ala 527, Ser 530
	Umbelliferone	3	-171.84	Ala 199, Ala 202, Gln 203, Thr 206, Tyr 385, Leu 391
	Indometacin	1	-280.13	Gln 192, Tyr 348, Val 349, Leu 352, Ser 353, Leu 359, Tyr 385, Val 523

(Table 6) cont.....

Name of the Biomarker	Name of the Compound	Details of H-bond interaction	Atomic contact Energy (ACE)	Amino acid residues on docked domains
		No. of bond	Values	
LOX (Lipooxygenase) (1YGE)	Carvone	2	-97.04	Leu 136, Tyr 137, Ser 139, Ser 168, Asp 181, Arg 182
	Limonene	0	-156.72	Ser 27, Ala 28, Val 29
	Umbelliferone	1	-145.51	Ala 28, Val 29, Met 103
	Indomethacin	5	-143.98	Tyr 137, Lys 138, Ser 139, Val 140, Ser 168, Tyr 180, Asp 181, Ile 183

Table 7. Docking sites and their atomic contact energy values for cancer.

Name of the Biomarker	Name of the Compound	Details of H-bond interaction	Atomic contact Energy (ACE)	Amino acid residues on docked domains
		No. of bond	Values	
p53-Mdm2 (4HFZ)	Carvone	0	-91.05	Phe 55, Gly 59, Trp 23, Lys 24
	Limonene	0	-92.75	Lys 24, Lys 51, Phe 55
	Umbelliferone	2	-90.52	Gln 24, Glu 25, Thr 26, Met 50, Lys 51
	Doxorubicin	7	-105.30	Gly 87, Val 88, Lys 98, Arg 105, Val 41, Gly 42, ala 43, Gln 44, Lys 45, Try 56, Gln 59
EGFR (epidermal growth factor receptor) (2GS2)	Carvone	1	-141.62	Leu 679, Arg 752, Leu 753
	Limonene	0	-135.95	Lys 721, Glu 722, Ala 726, Asn 732, Thr 761
	Umbelliferone	3	-130.31	Arg 752, Leu 753, Tyr 992
	Doxorubicin	9	-356.22	Asn 676, Gly 677, Ala 678, Leu 679, Arg 681, Leu 753

MOLECULAR DOCKING STUDIES

1. Stress Biomarkers

Symptoms are the major biomarkers for any disorder or disease that our body expresses. These symptoms progressively lead to stress conditions that activate the release of excess amounts of free radicals including reactive oxygen species. Anti-oxidant enzymes are the first line of defense against reactive oxygen species specifically superoxide dismutase [125]. Anti-oxidant enzymes such as superoxide dismutase, catalase, and glutathione peroxidase are the major biomarkers for targeting stress (Fig. **4**).

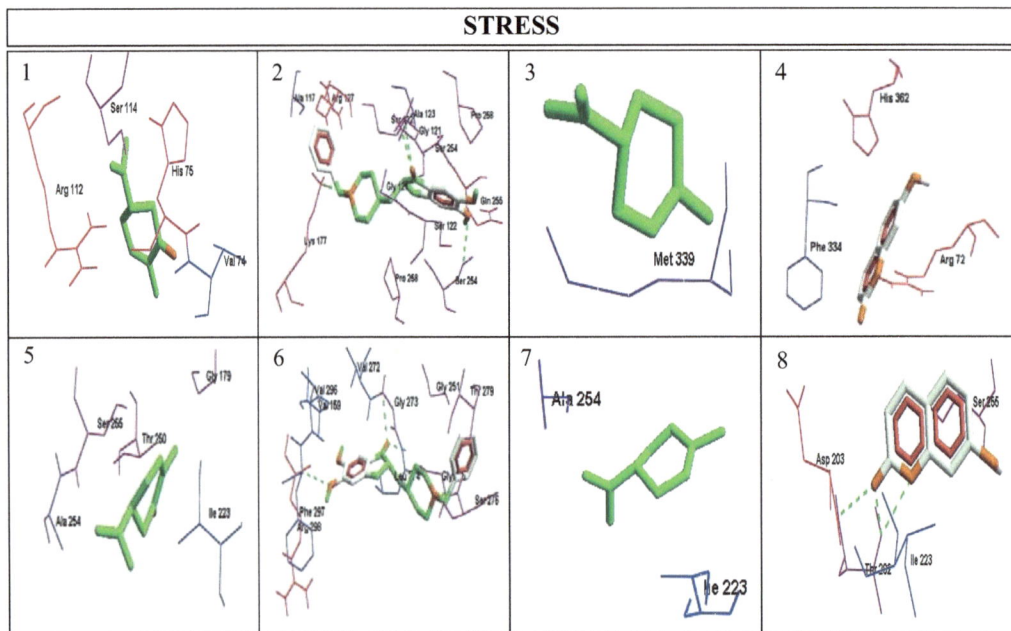

Fig. (4). (1) Catalase and Carvone, (2) Catalase and Limonene, (3) Catalase and Umbeliferone, (4) Catalase and Donazepril, (5) SOD and Carvone, (6) SOD and Limonene, (7) SOD, and Umbelliferone, (8) SOD and Donazepril.

Atomic contact energy values determine the bond energy or interaction between the molecules, the more the negative value greater is the interaction. The results demonstrated that limonene with catalase and umbelliferone with superoxide dismutase exhibited an ACE value of -144.54 and -147.66, respectively among the top 3 phytomolecules. The standard drug donazepril exhibited an ACE value of -250.63 with catalase and -365.13 with SOD, respectively (Table **5**). Since umbelliferone and limonene are natural phytomolecules these could be used as anti-stress agents as an alternative for the chemically synthesized drug in a dose-dependent manner.

2. Inflammation Biomarkers

The first defense molecules that play an essential role in the pathogenesis of inflammation are neutrophils. These molecules with the help of vascular endothelial cells travel to the extracellular space and release proteases, reactive oxygen species and chemokines [126]. Prolonged stressful conditions lead to inflammation causing injury to matrix proteins and normal tissues. The major biomarkers involved in inflammation (Fig. **5**) include cyclooxygenase-2 (COX) and lipooxygenase (LOX) [127].

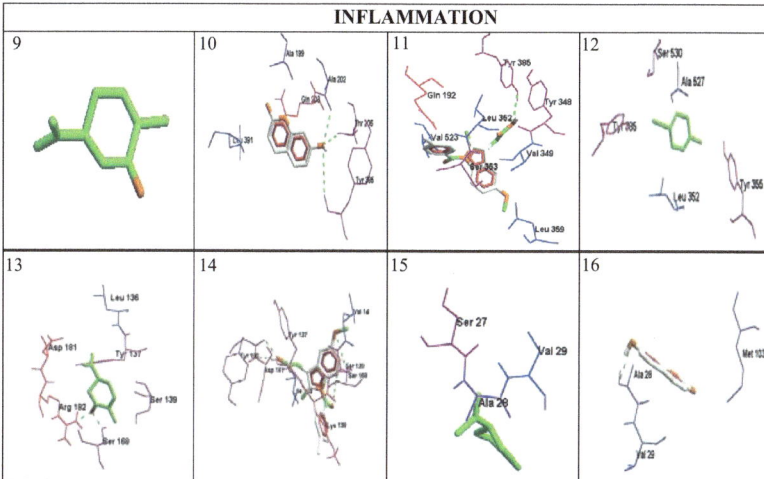

Fig. (5). (9) COX2 and Carvone, (10) COX2 and Limonene, (11) COX2 and Umbelliferone, (12) COX2 and Indomethacin, (13) LOX and Carvone, (14) LOX and Limonene, (15) LOX and Umbelliferone, (16) LOX and Indomethacin.

The results exhibited that umbelliferone with COX-2 and limonene with LOX has ACE values of -171.84 and -156.72, respectively among the top 3 phytomolecules. The standard drug Indomethacin has an ACE value -280.13 and -143.98, respectively (Table **6**).

3. Cancer Biomarkers

Globally cancer is the second most leading cause of death, the World Health Organization estimates that 9.6 million people worldwide would die of cancer and 12 million death would be the result by 2030 globally [128]. Depending on the stage of cancer the patients are treated through radiotherapy, hormonal ablation, chemotherapy and surgery [129]. Furthermore, treatment for cancer is very expensive and poor patients suffering from cancer will remain unaffordable. Lately, the use of herbs, shrubs have allured abundant attention as an alternative therapy for cancer for their lower toxicity and cost-effectiveness [130]. The major biomarkers involved in cancer include p53-Mdm2 and epidermal growth factor receptor (Fig. **6**).

Fig. (6). (17) p53-Mdm2 and Carvone, (18) p53-Mdm2 and Limonene, (19) p53-Mdm2 and Umbelliferone, (20) p53-Mdm2 and Doxorubicin, (21) EGFR and Carvone, (22) EGFR and Limonene, (23) EGFR and Umbelliferone, (24) EGFR and Doxorubicin.

The results exhibited that umbelliferone with p53-mdm2 and with EGFR has ACE values of -90.52 and -130.31, respectively among the top 3 phytomolecules. The standard drug doxorubicin has an ACE value of -105.30 and -356.22, respectively (Table **7**). On average umbelliferone isolated from dill seeds is one of the most potent phytomolecule based on the atomic contact energy values that were obtained from the structure-activity relationship studies (Tables **5, 6** & Table **7**) to treat a variety of diseases.

CONCLUSION

Ayurveda is one of the oldest systems of medicine that is one of India's historical roots. Ayurvedic medicines have been extensively used as a holistic approach to treat several diseases as alternative medicine. Dill seeds have been extensively used to treat gynecological disorders due to its exotic potential in Ayurveda but the mechanism of action and its pharmacology and pharmacodynamic properties still need to be explored. The chemical components responsible for ameliorating the diseases have to be determined. Formulation needs to be designed that can treat a group of diseases with the high potential ability and are cost-effective. Since Ayurveda only deals with formulations the efficacy of the crude will not provide satisfactory results, therefore understanding the chemistry of the phytomolecules, pharmacology, and mechanism of action needs to be deduced.

FUNDING

Dayananda Sagar University Seed Grant for Faculty Development was provided for the current research work. Further, the funding agency doesn't have any registry (the above mentioned is a university internal grant).

CONSENT FOR PUBLICATION

Not applicable.

CONFLICT OF INTERESTS

The authors declare no conflict of interest, financial or otherwise.

ACKNOWLEDGMENTS

Dr. Kounaina Khan and Prof. SP Hudeda thank JSS Ayurvedic Medical College and Hospital for the encouragement and support provided during the preparation of the book chapter. Dr. Farhan Zameer, sincerely acknowledges the University Grants Commission (UGC), Govt. of India, New Delhi, for awarding Raman Post-Doctoral Fellowship to USA (Ref No. F.5-97/2014 (IC) FD dairy no: 6725). Mr. Pankaj Satapathy would like to thank DST-KSTePS, GoK, for providing DST Ph.D. fellowship (LIF-09-2018-19). Further, we extend our gratitude towards the management and office bearers of Dayananda Sagar University, Bengaluru, Karnataka, India, for constant inspiration, motivation, and encouragement to pursue scientific research.

REFERENCES

[1]   Dhanvantari nighuntu, edited by Prof. P.V. Sharma and translated by Dr. G. R. Sharma, Published by Chaukhambha orientalia, Varanasi 2nd edition, 1998, Shatapushpadi varga/1.

[2]   Warrier PK, Nambiar VPK, Ramakutty C. Arya Vaidya Sala. Kottakkal Madras, India: Orient Longman Limited 1994; 1: pp. 153-4. Indian Medicinal Plants

[3]   Santos PA, Figueiredo AC, Lourenço PM, *et al.* Hairy root cultures of *Anethum Graveolens* (dill): establishment, growth, time-course study of their essential oil and its comparison with parent plant oils. Biotechnol Lett 2002; 24(12): 1031-6.
      [http://dx.doi.org/10.1023/A:1015653701265]

[4]   Carrubba A, La Torre R, Saiano F, Aiello P. Sustainable production of fennel and dill by intercropping. Agron Sustain Dev 2008; 28(2): 247-56.
      [http://dx.doi.org/10.1051/agro:2007040]

[5]   Wanner H, Gu H, Dorn S. Nutritional value of floral nectar sources for flight in the parasitoid wasp, *Cotesia glomerata.* Physiol Entomol 2006; 31(2): 127-33.
      [http://dx.doi.org/10.1111/j.1365-3032.2006.00494.x]

[6]   Jana S, Shekhawat GS. *Anethum Graveolens*: An Indian traditional medicinal herb and spice. Pharmacogn Rev 2010; 4(8): 179-84.
      [http://dx.doi.org/10.4103/0973-7847.70915] [PMID: 22228959]

[7]   Bouwmeester HJ, Gershenzon J, Konings MC, Croteau R. Biosynthesis of the monoterpenes limonene and carvone in the fruit of caraway. I. Demonstration Of enzyme activities and their changes with development. Plant Physiol 1998; 117(3): 901-12.
[http://dx.doi.org/10.1104/pp.117.3.901] [PMID: 9662532]

[8]   Ayurvedic Pharmacopoeia of India, published by ministry of health and family welfare. 1. 2003; II: p. 15.

[9]   Kirtikar KR, Basu BD. Indian medicinal plants. Indian Medicinal Plants 1935.

[10]   Whiting DR, Guariguata L, Weil C, Shaw J. IDF diabetes atlas: global estimates of the prevalence of diabetes for 2011 and 2030. Diabetes Res Clin Pract 2011; 94(3): 311-21.
[http://dx.doi.org/10.1016/j.diabres.2011.10.029] [PMID: 22079683]

[11]   Wild S, Roglic G, Green A, Sicree R, King H. Global prevalence of diabetes: Estimates for the year 2000 and projections for 2030. Diabetes Care 2004; 27(5): 1047-53.
[http://dx.doi.org/10.2337/diacare.27.5.1047] [PMID: 15111519]

[12]   Liao JK. HDL cholesterol, very low levels of LDL cholesterol, and cardiovascular events. Curr Atheroscler Rep 2008; 10(4): 281.
[http://dx.doi.org/10.1007/s11883-008-0043-x] [PMID: 18606093]

[13]   Van Olmen J, Schellevis F, Van Damme W, Kegels G, Rasschaert F. Management of chronic diseases in sub-Saharan Africa: cross-fertilisation between HIV/AIDS and diabetes care. J of trop med 2012; 2012

[14]   Shahryari J, Poormorteza M, Noori-Sorkhani A, Divsalar K, Abbasi-Oshaghi E. The effect of concomitant ethanol and opium consumption on lipid profiles and atherosclerosis in golden syrian Hamster's aorta. Addict Health 2013; 5(3-4): 83-9.
[PMID: 24494163]

[15]   Taghi GM, Mohsen R, Hossein P, Saied A. Effect of *in vitro* glycation of human placental collagen (Type IV) on platelet aggregation. Pak J Biol Sci 2005; 8: 1203-6.
[http://dx.doi.org/10.3923/pjbs.2005.1203.1206]

[16]   Lubitz I, Ricny J, Atrakchi-Baranes D, *et al.* High dietary advanced glycation end products are associated with poorer spatial learning and accelerated Aβ deposition in an Alzheimer mouse model. Aging Cell 2016; 15(2): 309-16.
[http://dx.doi.org/10.1111/acel.12436] [PMID: 26781037]

[17]   Maritim AC, Sanders RA, Watkins JB III. Diabetes, oxidative stress, and antioxidants: A review. J Biochem Mol Toxicol 2003; 17(1): 24-38.
[http://dx.doi.org/10.1002/jbt.10058] [PMID: 12616644]

[18]   Mohammadi A, Mirzaei F, Jamshidi M, *et al.* The *In Vivo* biochemical and oxidative changes by ethanol and opium consumption in Syrian hamsters. Int J Biol 2013; 5(4): 14.
[http://dx.doi.org/10.5539/ijb.v5n4p14]

[19]   Rahimi R, Nikfar S, Larijani B, Abdollahi M. A review on the role of antioxidants in the management of diabetes and its complications. Biomed Pharmacother 2005; 59(7): 365-73.
[http://dx.doi.org/10.1016/j.biopha.2005.07.002] [PMID: 16081237]

[20]   Mirzaeipour F, Azdaki N, Mohammadi GA. The effects of opium addiction through different administration routes on inflammatory and coagulation factors. J Kerman Univ Med Sci 2013; 20(3)

[21]   Somsak V, Chachiyo S, Jaihan U, Nakinchat S. Protective effect of aqueous crude extract of neem (Azadirachta indica) leaves on Plasmodium berghei-induced renal damage in mice. Journal of trop med 2015; 2015

[22]   Alvarez-Uria G, Midde M, Pakam R, Yalla PS, Naik PK, Reddy R. Short-course induction treatment with intrathecal amphotericin B lipid emulsion for HIV infected patients with cryptococcal meningitis. Journal of tropical medicine 2015; 2015

[http://dx.doi.org/10.1155/2015/864271]

[23] Mohammadi A, Norouzian P, Jamshidi M, Najafi N, Oshaghi EA. Effect of garlic (*Allium sativum*) on lipid profiles, antioxidant activity and expression of scavenger receptor class B type I (SR-BI) in liver and intestine of hypercholesterolemic mice. Journal. J of Adv in Chem 2013; 5(3)
[http://dx.doi.org/10.24297/jac.v5i3.2665]

[24] Yazdanparast R, Bahramikia S. Evaluation of the effect of *Anethum Graveolens* L. crude extracts on serum lipids and lipoproteins profiles in hypercholesterolaemic rats. Daru 2008; 16(2): 88-94.

[25] Goodarzi MT, Khodadadi I, Tavilani H, Abbasi Oshaghi E. The role of *Anethum Graveolens* L.(Dill) in the management of diabetes. Journal of tropical medicine 2016; 2016

[26] Panda S. The effect of *Anethum Graveolens* L. (dill) on corticosteroid induced diabetes mellitus: involvement of thyroid hormones. Phytother Res 2008; 22(12): 1695-7.
[http://dx.doi.org/10.1002/ptr.2553] [PMID: 18814208]

[27] Yalcin MM, Altinova AE, Ozkan C, *et al.* Thyroid malignancy risk of incidental thyroid nodules in patients with non-thyroid cancer. Acta Endocrinol (Bucur) 2016; 12(2): 185-90.
[http://dx.doi.org/10.4183/aeb.2016.185] [PMID: 31149085]

[28] Rashidi AA, Mirhashemi SM, Taghizadeh M, Sarkhail P. Iranian medicinal plants for diabetes mellitus: a systematic review. Pak J Biol Sci 2013; 16(9): 401-11.
[http://dx.doi.org/10.3923/pjbs.2013.401.411] [PMID: 24498803]

[29] Idiz C, Aysan E, Elmas L, Bahadori F, Idiz UO. Effectiveness of *Anethum Graveolens* l. On antioxidant status, thyroid function and histopathology. Acta Endocrinol (Bucur) 2018; 14(4): 447-52.
[http://dx.doi.org/10.4183/aeb.2018.447] [PMID: 31149295]

[30] Milionis HJ, Rizos E, Goudevenos J, Seferiadis K, Mikhailidis DP, Elisaf MS. Components of the metabolic syndrome and risk for first-ever acute ischemic nonembolic stroke in elderly subjects. Stroke 2005; 36(7): 1372-6.
[http://dx.doi.org/10.1161/01.STR.0000169935.35394.38] [PMID: 15933255]

[31] Nys GM, van Zandvoort MJ, de Kort PL, Jansen BP, Kappelle LJ, de Haan EH. Restrictions of the Mini-Mental State Examination in acute stroke. Arch Clin Neuropsychol 2005; 20(5): 623-9.
[http://dx.doi.org/10.1016/j.acn.2005.04.001] [PMID: 15939186]

[32] Kawvised S, Wattanathorn J, Thukham-mee W. Neuroprotective and cognitive-enhancing effects of microencapsulation of mulberry fruit extract in an animal model of menopausal women with metabolic syndrome. Oxidative medicine and cellular longevity 2017; 2017
[http://dx.doi.org/10.1155/2017/2962316]

[33] Mesripour A, Rafieian-Kopaei M, Bahrami B. The effects of *Anethum Graveolens* essence on scopolamine-induced memory impairment in mice. Res Pharm Sci 2016; 11(2): 145-51.
[PMID: 27168754]

[34] Beulah KC, Aishwarya T. Screening for bioactives from Indian medicinal herbs – a simplistic approach for antioxidant metabolites. Int J Pharm Pharm Sci 2015; 7(1): 195-8.

[35] Limtrakul P, Yodkeeree S, Pitchakarn P, Punfa W. Anti-inflammatory effects of proanthocyanidin-rich red rice extract *via* suppression of MAPK, AP-1 and NF-κB pathways in Raw 264.7 macrophages. Nutr Res Pract 2016; 10(3): 251-8.
[http://dx.doi.org/10.4162/nrp.2016.10.3.251] [PMID: 27247720]

[36] Ohnon W, Wattanathorn J, Thukham-mee W, Muchimapura S, Wannanon P, Tong-un T. The Combined Extract of Black Sticky Rice and Dill Improves Poststroke Cognitive Impairment in Metabolic Syndrome Condition. Oxidative medicine and cellular longevity 2019; 2019
[http://dx.doi.org/10.1155/2019/9089035]

[37] Trefts E, Gannon M, Wasserman DH. The liver. Curr Biol 2017; 27(21): R1147-51.
[http://dx.doi.org/10.1016/j.cub.2017.09.019] [PMID: 29112863]

[38] Corey KE, Chalasani N. Management of dyslipidemia as a cardiovascular risk factor in individuals with nonalcoholic fatty liver disease. Clin Gastroenterol Hepatol 2014; 12(7): 1077-84.
[http://dx.doi.org/10.1016/j.cgh.2013.08.014] [PMID: 23962548]

[39] Abbasi Oshaghi E, Khodadadi I, Saidijam M, *et al.* Lipid lowering effects of hydroalcoholic extract of *Anethum Graveolens* L. and dill tablet in high cholesterol fed hamsters. Cholesterol 2015; 2015

[40] Kumar V, Abbas AK, Aster JC. Robbins basic pathology e-book. Elsevier Health Sciences 2017.

[41] Hosseinzadeh H, Ramezani M, Salmani G. Antinociceptive, anti-inflammatory and acute toxicity effects of *Zataria multiflora* Boiss extracts in mice and rats. J Ethnopharmacol 2000; 73(3): 379-85.
[http://dx.doi.org/10.1016/S0378-8741(00)00238-5] [PMID: 11090990]

[42] Delaquis PJ, Stanich K, Girard B, Mazza G. Antimicrobial activity of individual and mixed fractions of dill, cilantro, coriander and eucalyptus essential oils. Int J Food Microbiol 2002; 74(1-2): 101-9.
[http://dx.doi.org/10.1016/S0168-1605(01)00734-6] [PMID: 11929164]

[43] Selen Isbilir S, Sagiroglu A. Antioxidant potential of different Dill (*Anethum Graveolens* L.) leaf extracts. Int J Food Prop 2011; 14(4): 894-902.
[http://dx.doi.org/10.1080/10942910903474401]

[44] Ravindra S. Agro-techniques of medicinal plants. Daya Publishing House 2004.

[45] Pullaiah T. Medicinal plants in India. Daya Books 2002.

[46] Duke JA. Handbook of medicinal herbs. CRC Press 2002.
[http://dx.doi.org/10.1201/9781420040463]

[47] Naseri M, Mojab F, Khodadoost M, *et al.* The study of anti-inflammatory activity of oil-based dill (*Anethum Graveolens* L.) extract used topically in formalin-induced inflammation male rat paw. Iranian journal of pharmaceutical research. Iran J Pharm Res 2012; 11(4): 1169-74.
[PMID: 24250550]

[48] Ma JS, Kim WJ, Kim JJ, *et al.* Gold nanoparticles attenuate LPS-induced NO production through the inhibition of NF-kappaB and IFN-β/STAT1 pathways in RAW264.7 cells. Nitric Oxide 2010; 23(3): 214-9.
[http://dx.doi.org/10.1016/j.niox.2010.06.005] [PMID: 20547236]

[49] Ghosh S, May MJ, Kopp EB. NF-κ B and Rel proteins: evolutionarily conserved mediators of immune responses. Annu Rev Immunol 1998; 16(1): 225-60.
[http://dx.doi.org/10.1146/annurev.immunol.16.1.225] [PMID: 9597130]

[50] Detmers PA, Hernandez M, Mudgett J, *et al.* Deficiency in inducible nitric oxide synthase results in reduced atherosclerosis in apolipoprotein E-deficient mice. J Immunol 2000; 165(6): 3430-5.
[http://dx.doi.org/10.4049/jimmunol.165.6.3430] [PMID: 10975863]

[51] Chan ED, Riches DW. IFN-γ + LPS induction of iNOS is modulated by ERK, JNK/SAPK, and p38-MAPK in a mouse macrophage cell line. Am J Physiol Cell Physiol 2001; 280(3): C441-50.
[http://dx.doi.org/10.1152/ajpcell.2001.280.3.C441] [PMID: 11171562]

[52] Kim YJ, Shin Y, Lee KH, Kim TJ. *Anethum graveloens* flower extracts inhibited a lipopolysaccharide-induced inflammatory response by blocking iNOS expression and NF-κB activity in macrophages. Biosci Biotechnol Biochem 2012; 76(6): 1122-7.
[http://dx.doi.org/10.1271/bbb.110950] [PMID: 22790933]

[53] 2002.

[54] Pham-Huy LA, He H, Pham-Huy C. Free radicals, antioxidants in disease and health. Int J Biomed Sci 2008; 4(2): 89-96.
[PMID: 23675073]

[55] Battin EE, Brumaghim JL. Antioxidant activity of sulfur and selenium: a review of reactive oxygen species scavenging, glutathione peroxidase, and metal-binding antioxidant mechanisms. Cell Biochem

Biophys 2009; 55(1): 1-23.
[http://dx.doi.org/10.1007/s12013-009-9054-7] [PMID: 19548119]

[56] Oshaghi EA, Khodadadi I, Mirzaei F, Khazaei M, Tavilani H, Goodarzi MT. methanolic extract of dill leaves inhibits AGEs formation and shows potential hepatoprotective effects in CCl4 Induced liver toxicity in rats. Journal of pharmaceutics 2017; 2017

[57] Li Z, Xue Y, Li M, *et al.* The Antioxidation of Different Fractions of Dill (*Anethum Graveolens*) and Their Influences on Cytokines in Macrophages RAW264.7. J Oleo Sci 2018; 67(12): 1535-41.
[http://dx.doi.org/10.5650/jos.ess18134] [PMID: 30429445]

[58] Porsolt RD, Le Pichon M, Jalfre M. Depression: a new animal model sensitive to antidepressant treatments. Nature 1977; 266(5604): 730-2.
[http://dx.doi.org/10.1038/266730a0] [PMID: 559941]

[59] El Mansouri L, Bousta D, El Youbi-El Hamsas A, Boukhira S, Akdime H. Phytochemical screening, antidepressant and analgesic effects of aqueous extract of *Anethum Graveolens* L. from southeast of Morocco. Am J Ther 2016; 23(6): e1695-9.
[http://dx.doi.org/10.1097/MJT.0000000000000090] [PMID: 26872137]

[60] Orhan I, Kusmenoglu S, Sener B. GC-MS analysis of the seed oil of *Cannabis sativa* L. cultivated in Turkey. Eczacilik Fakultesi Dergisi-Gazi Universitesi 2000; 17(2): 79-82.

[61] Singh G, Maurya S, De Lampasona MP, Catalan C. Chemical constituents, antimicrobial investigations, and antioxidative potentials of *Anethum Graveolens* L. essential oil and acetone extract: Part 52. J Food Sci 2005; 70(4): M208-15.
[http://dx.doi.org/10.1111/j.1365-2621.2005.tb07190.x]

[62] Saini N, Singh GK, Nagori BP. Spasmolytic potential of some medicinal plants belonging to family Umbelliferae: a review. Int J Res Ayurveda Pharm 2014; 5(1): 74-83.
[http://dx.doi.org/10.7897/2277-4343.05116]

[63] Vispute MM, Sharma D, Mandal AB, Rokade JJ, Tyagi PK, Yadav AS. Effect of dietary supplementation of hemp (*Cannabis sativa*) and dill seed (*Anethum Graveolens*) on performance, serum biochemicals and gut health of broiler chickens. J Anim Physiol Anim Nutr (Berl) 2019; 103(2): 525-33.
[http://dx.doi.org/10.1111/jpn.13052] [PMID: 30604902]

[64] McCormack TT, Sims J, Eyre-Brook I, *et al.* Gastric lesions in portal hypertension: inflammatory gastritis or congestive gastropathy? Gut 1985; 26(11): 1226-32.
[http://dx.doi.org/10.1136/gut.26.11.1226] [PMID: 3877665]

[65] Alvarez A, Pomar F, Sevilla MA, Montero MJ. Gastric antisecretory and antiulcer activities of an ethanolic extract of *Bidens pilosa L. var. radiata Schult.* Bip. J Ethnopharmacol 1999; 67(3): 333-40.
[http://dx.doi.org/10.1016/S0378-8741(99)00092-6] [PMID: 10617069]

[66] Hosseinzadeh H, Karimi GR, Ameri M. Effects of *Anethum Graveolens* L. seed extracts on experimental gastric irritation models in mice. BMC Pharmacol 2002; 2(1): 21
[http://dx.doi.org/10.1186/1471-2210-2-21] [PMID: 12493079]

[67] Salyers AA, Whitt DD, Whitt DD. Bacterial pathogenesis: a molecular approach. Washington, DC: ASM press 1994.

[68] Chopra I, Hodgson J, Metcalf B, Poste G. The search for antimicrobial agents effective against bacteria resistant to multiple antibiotics. Antimicrob Agents Chemother 1997; 41(3): 497-503.
[http://dx.doi.org/10.1128/AAC.41.3.497] [PMID: 9055982]

[69] Evans WC. Trease and Evans pharmagognosy. 15th ed., London: Elsevier Sci Ltd 2002.

[70] Kaur GJ, Arora DS. Antibacterial and phytochemical screening of *Anethum Graveolens*, Foeniculum vulgare and *Trachyspermum ammi*. BMC Complement Altern Med 2009; 9(1): 30.
[http://dx.doi.org/10.1186/1472-6882-9-30] [PMID: 19656417]

[71]   Manefield M, Rasmussen TB, Henzter M, *et al.* Halogenated furanones inhibit quorum sensing through accelerated LuxR turnover. Microbiology 2002; 148(Pt 4): 1119-27.
[http://dx.doi.org/10.1099/00221287-148-4-1119] [PMID: 11932456]

[72]   Packiavathy IA, Agilandeswari P, Musthafa KS, Pandian SK, Ravi AV. Antibiofilm and quorum sensing inhibitory potential of *Cuminum cyminum* and its secondary metabolite methyl eugenol against Gram-negative bacterial pathogens. Food Res Int 2012; 45(1): 85-92.
[http://dx.doi.org/10.1016/j.foodres.2011.10.022]

[73]   Meghashri. S, Chauhan. JB, Syed. AA and Farhan Zameer. Effect of *Ocimum tenuiflorum* leaf extract against infective endocarditis. Int J Phytomed 2011; 3(4): 470-4.

[74]   Salini R, Pandian SK. Interference of quorum sensing in urinary pathogen *Serratia marcescens* by *Anethum Graveolens*. Pathog Dis 2015; 73(6)ftv038
[http://dx.doi.org/10.1093/femspd/ftv038] [PMID: 26013821]

[75]   Vallabhaneni S, Mody RK, Walker T, Chiller T. The global burden of fungal diseases. Infect Dis Clin North Am 2016; 30(1): 1-11.
[http://dx.doi.org/10.1016/j.idc.2015.10.004] [PMID: 26739604]

[76]   Pereira Gonzales F, Maisch T. Photodynamic inactivation for controlling *Candida albicans* infections. Fungal Biol 2012; 116(1): 1-10.
[http://dx.doi.org/10.1016/j.funbio.2011.10.001] [PMID: 22208597]

[77]   Chen Y, Zeng H, Tian J, Ban X, Ma B, Wang Y. Antifungal mechanism of essential oil from *Anethum Graveolens* seeds against *Candida albicans*. J Med Microbiol 2013; 62(Pt 8): 1175-83.
[http://dx.doi.org/10.1099/jmm.0.055467-0] [PMID: 23657528]

[78]   Chen Y, Zeng H, Tian J, Ban X, Ma B, Wang Y. Dill (*Anethum Graveolens* L.) seed essential oil induces Candida albicans apoptosis in a metacaspase-dependent manner. Fungal Biol 2014; 118(4): 394-401.
[http://dx.doi.org/10.1016/j.funbio.2014.02.004] [PMID: 24742834]

[79]   Barber BE, Rajahram GS, Grigg MJ, William T, Anstey NM. World Malaria Report: time to acknowledge *Plasmodium knowlesi* malaria. Malar J 2017; 16(1): 135.
[http://dx.doi.org/10.1186/s12936-017-1787-y] [PMID: 28359340]

[80]   Soltani A, Vatandoost H, Oshaghi MA, Ravasan NM, Enayati AA, Asgarian F. Resistance mechanisms of *Anopheles stephensi* (Diptera: Culicidae) to temephos. J Arthropod Borne Dis 2014; 9(1): 71-83.
[PMID: 26114145]

[81]   Govindarajan M, Rajeswary M, Senthilmurugan S, *et al.* Curzerene, trans-β-elemenone, and γ-elemene as effective larvicides against *Anopheles subpictus, Aedes albopictus*, and *Culex tritaeniorhynchus*: toxicity on non-target aquatic predators. Environ Sci Pollut Res Int 2018; 25(11): 10272-82.
[http://dx.doi.org/10.1007/s11356-017-8822-y] [PMID: 28353108]

[82]   Osanloo M, Sereshti H, Sedaghat MM, Amani A. Nanoemulsion of Dill essential oil as a green and potent larvicide against *Anopheles stephensi*. Environ Sci Pollut Res Int 2018; 25(7): 6466-73.
[http://dx.doi.org/10.1007/s11356-017-0822-4] [PMID: 29250730]

[83]   Monsefi M, Ghasemi M, Bahaoddini A. The effects of *Anethum Graveolens* L. on female reproductive system of rats. Daru 2006; 14(3): 131-5.

[84]   Malihezaman M, Mojaba M, Elham H, Farnaz G, Ramin M. Anti-fertility effects of different fractions of *Anethum Graveolens* L. extracts on female rats. Afr J Tradit Complement Altern Med 2012; 9(3): 336-41.
[http://dx.doi.org/10.4314/ajtcam.v9i3.6] [PMID: 23983364]

[85]   Monsefi M, Zahmati M, Masoudi M, Javidnia K. Effects of *Anethum Graveolens* L. on fertility in male rats. Eur J Contracept Reprod Health Care 2011; 16(6): 488-97.
[http://dx.doi.org/10.3109/13625187.2011.622815] [PMID: 22066892]

[86]   Monsefi M, Khalifeh B, Nikeghbal S. Effects of *Anethum Graveolens* L. on *In Vitro* Matured Mouse Oocytes and Granulosa Cells. Avicenna J Med Biotechnol 2018; 10(4): 220-6.
[PMID: 30555654]

[87]   Modarresi M, Farahpour MR, Baradaran B. Topical application of *Mentha piperita* essential oil accelerates wound healing in infected mice model. Inflammopharmacology 2019; 27(3): 531-7.
[http://dx.doi.org/10.1007/s10787-018-0510-0] [PMID: 29980963]

[88]   Jiang L, Dai Y, Cui F, *et al.* Expression of cytokines, growth factors and apoptosis-related signal molecules in chronic pressure ulcer wounds healing. Spinal Cord 2014; 52(2): 145-51.
[http://dx.doi.org/10.1038/sc.2013.132] [PMID: 24296807]

[89]   Berridge MJ. Module 11: cell stress, inflammatory responses and cell death. Cell Signaling Biology 2014; 6csb0001011
[http://dx.doi.org/10.1042/csb0001011]

[90]   Li F, Huang Q, Chen J, *et al.* Apoptotic cells activate the "phoenix rising" pathway to promote wound healing and tissue regeneration. Sci Signal 2010; 3(110): ra13.
[http://dx.doi.org/10.1126/scisignal.2000634] [PMID: 20179271]

[91]   Manzuoerh R, Farahpour MR, Oryan A, Sonboli A. Effectiveness of topical administration of *Anethum Graveolens* essential oil on MRSA-infected wounds. Biomed Pharmacother 2019; 109: 1650-8.
[http://dx.doi.org/10.1016/j.biopha.2018.10.117] [PMID: 30551419]

[92]   Food, Nutrition, Physical Activity, and the Prevention of Cancer: a Global Perspective. Washington, DC: American Institute for Cancer Research 2007.

[93]   Choo SP, Tan WL, Goh BKP, Tai WM, Zhu AX. Comparison of hepatocellular carcinoma in Eastern versus Western populations. Cancer 2016; 122(22): 3430-46.
[http://dx.doi.org/10.1002/cncr.30237] [PMID: 27622302]

[94]   Liu CY, Chen KF, Chen PJ. Treatment of liver cancer. Cold Spring Harb Perspect Med 2015; 5(9)a021535
[http://dx.doi.org/10.1101/cshperspect.a021535] [PMID: 26187874]

[95]   Malvika S, Satyapal S, Lal JM, Mita K. An Ayurveda approach to combat toxicity of chemo-radiotherapy in cancer patients. Int J Res Ayurveda Pharm 2016; 7 (Suppl. 2): 124-9.
[http://dx.doi.org/10.7897/2277-4343.07271]

[96]   Shah U, Shah R, Acharya S, Acharya N. Novel anticancer agents from plant sources. Chin J Nat Med 2013; 11(1): 16-23.
[http://dx.doi.org/10.3724/SP.J.1009.2013.00016]

[97]   Tariq A, Sadia S, Pan K, *et al.* A systematic review on ethnomedicines of anti-cancer plants. Phytother Res 2017; 31(2): 202-64.
[http://dx.doi.org/10.1002/ptr.5751] [PMID: 28093828]

[98]   Mohammed FA, Elkady AI, Syed FQ, Mirza MB, Hakeem KR, Alkarim S. *Anethum Graveolens* (dill) - A medicinal herb induces apoptosis and cell cycle arrest in HepG2 cell line. J Ethnopharmacol 2018; 219: 15-22.
[http://dx.doi.org/10.1016/j.jep.2018.03.008] [PMID: 29530611]

[99]   Hellard ME, Sinclair MI, Hogg GG, Fairley CK. Prevalence of enteric pathogens among community based asymptomatic individuals. J Gastroenterol Hepatol 2000; 15(3): 290-3.
[http://dx.doi.org/10.1046/j.1440-1746.2000.02089.x] [PMID: 10764030]

[100] Xiao L, Fayer R. Molecular characterisation of species and genotypes of Cryptosporidium and Giardia and assessment of zoonotic transmission. Int J Parasitol 2008; 38(11): 1239-55.
[http://dx.doi.org/10.1016/j.ijpara.2008.03.006] [PMID: 18479685]

[101] Lemée V, Zaharia I, Nevez G, *et al.* Metronidazole and albendazole susceptibility of 11 clinical

isolates of *Giardia duodenalis* from France. J Antimicrob Chemother 2000; 46(5): 819-21.
[http://dx.doi.org/10.1093/jac/46.5.819] [PMID: 11062206]

[102] Madhusudan M. Contribution of *Withania somnifera* against Platelet Aggregation and Inflammatory Enzymes and Screening of Bioactives by Molecular Docking. Pharm Biol 2015; 54(9): 1-6.

[103] Qu F, Zhou J. Electro-acupuncture in relieving labor pain. Evid Based Complement Alternat Med 2007; 4(1): 125-30.
[http://dx.doi.org/10.1093/ecam/nel053] [PMID: 17342250]

[104] Cheng YW, Hopkins LM, Laros RK Jr, Caughey AB. Duration of the second stage of labor in multiparous women: maternal and neonatal outcomes. Am J Obstet Gynecol 2007; 196(6): 585.e1-6.
[http://dx.doi.org/10.1016/j.ajog.2007.03.021] [PMID: 17547906]

[105] Hekmatzadeh SF, Bazarganipour F, Malekzadeh J, Goodarzi F, Aramesh S. A randomized clinical trial of the efficacy of applying a simple protocol of boiled *Anethum Graveolens* seeds on pain intensity and duration of labor stages. Complement Ther Med 2014; 22(6): 970-6.
[http://dx.doi.org/10.1016/j.ctim.2014.10.007] [PMID: 25453516]

[106] Charaka Samhita of Agnivesha. Chikitsa Sthana, chapter 14, shloka 41edition by Acharya Vidyadhara Shukla and Prof Ravi Dutt Tripathi, Chaukhamba Sanskrit Pratishthan, Delhi. 2007.

[107] Charaka Samhita of Agnivesha. vol 2, Chikitsa Sthana, chapter 29, shloka 140edition by Acharya Vidyadhara Shukla and Prof Ravi Dutt Tripathi, Chaukhamba Sanskrit Pratishthan, Delhi 2007.

[108] Shatapushpashatavari Kalpadhyaya, chapter 5, Shloka 19edited by Prof PV Tiwari, edition reprint 2002, Chaukhamba Vishvabharati, Varanasi. 2002.

[109] Samhita Kashyapa. Vidhyotini Hindi commentary by Shri Satyapala bhishagacharya. Dehli: Chaukambha publication 2013. Shatapushpashatavari Kalpadhyaya, P.N. 186.

[110] Sharma PC, Yelne MB, Dennis TJ. Database on medicinal plants used in Ayurveda, CCRAS, Dept of AYUSH, Ministry of Health and Family Welfare, Govt of India 2008; 8: 360.

[111] Hosseinzadeh H, Karimi GR, Ameri M. Effects of *Anethum Graveolens* L. seed extracts on experimental gastric irritation models in mice. BMC Pharmacol 2002; 2: 21.
[http://dx.doi.org/10.1186/1471-2210-2-21] [PMID: 12493079]

[112] Fleming T. PDR for Herbal Medicines. Medical Economics Company, New Jersy PN 2000; 252-3.

[113] Arora DS, Kaur JG. Antibacterial activity of some Indian medicinal plants. J Nat Med 2007; 61: 313-7.
[http://dx.doi.org/10.1007/s11418-007-0137-8]

[114] Ding X, Chen H. Anticancer effects of Carvone in myeloma cells is mediated through the inhibition of p38 MAPK signaling pathway, apoptosis induction and inhibition of cell invasion. Journal of BU ON: official journal of the Balkan Union of Oncology 2018; 23(3): 747-51.

[115] Bacanlı M, Başaran AA, Başaran N. The antioxidant and antigenotoxic properties of citrus phenolics limonene and naringin. Food Chem Toxicol 2015; 81: 160-70.
[http://dx.doi.org/10.1016/j.fct.2015.04.015] [PMID: 25896273]

[116] Pan L, Li X, Jin H, Yang X, Qin B. Antifungal activity of umbelliferone derivatives: Synthesis and structure-activity relationships. Microb Pathog 2017; 104: 110-5.
[http://dx.doi.org/10.1016/j.micpath.2017.01.024] [PMID: 28089948]

[117] Ramu R, S Shirahatti P, S NS, Zameer F, Bl D, M N NP. Correction: Assessment of *In Vivo* Antidiabetic Properties of Umbelliferone and Lupeol Constituents of Banana (*Musa* sp. var. Nanjangud Rasa Bale) Flower in Hyperglycaemic Rodent Model. PLoS One 2016; 11(7)e0160048
[http://dx.doi.org/10.1371/journal.pone.0160048] [PMID: 27438346]

[118] Ramu R, Shirahatti PS, Nayakavadi S, *et al.* The effect of a plant extract enriched in stigmasterol and β-sitosterol on glycaemic status and glucose metabolism in alloxan-induced diabetic rats. Food Funct 2016; 7(9): 3999-4011.

[http://dx.doi.org/10.1039/C6FO00343E] [PMID: 27711824]

[119] Ramu R, Shirahatti PS, Anilakumar KR, *et al.* Assessment of nutritional quality and global antioxidant response of banana (*Musa sp. CV. Nanjangud Rasa Bale*) pseudostem and flower. Pharmacognosy Res 2017; 9 (Suppl. 1): S74-83.
[http://dx.doi.org/10.4103/pr.pr_67_17] [PMID: 29333047]

[120] Ramu R, Shirahatti PS, Zameer F, Prasad MN. Investigation of antihyperglycaemic activity of banana (*Musa sp. var. Nanjangud rasa bale*) pseudostem in normal and diabetic rats. J Sci Food Agric 2015; 95(1): 165-73.
[http://dx.doi.org/10.1002/jsfa.6698] [PMID: 24752944]

[121] Lee HR, Kim GH, Choi WS, Park IK. Repellent activity of *Apiaceae* plant essential oils and their constituents against adult German cockroaches. J Econ Entomol 2017; 110(2): 552-7.
[http://dx.doi.org/10.1093/jee/tow290] [PMID: 28165121]

[122] Sahib AS, Mohammed IH, Sloo SA. Antigiardial effect of *Anethum Graveolens* aqueous extract in children. J Intercult Ethnopharmacol 2014; 3(3): 109-12.
[http://dx.doi.org/10.5455/jice.20140523104104] [PMID: 26401357]

[123] Thomsen R, Christensen MH. MolDock: a new technique for high-accuracy molecular docking. J Med Chem 2006; 49(11): 3315-21.
[http://dx.doi.org/10.1021/jm051197e] [PMID: 16722650]

[124] Schüttelkopf AW, van Aalten DM. PRODRG: a tool for high-throughput crystallography of protein-ligand complexes. Acta Crystallogr D Biol Crystallogr 2004; 60(Pt 8): 1355-63.
[http://dx.doi.org/10.1107/S0907444904011679] [PMID: 15272157]

[125] Landis GN, Tower J. Superoxide dismutase evolution and life span regulation. Mech Ageing Dev 2005; 126(3): 365-79.
[http://dx.doi.org/10.1016/j.mad.2004.08.012] [PMID: 15664623]

[126] Yasui K, Baba A. Therapeutic potential of superoxide dismutase (SOD) for resolution of inflammation. Inflamm Res 2006; 55(9): 359-63.
[http://dx.doi.org/10.1007/s00011-006-5195-y] [PMID: 17122956]

[127] Seibert K, Masferrer JL. Role of inducible cyclooxygenase (COX-2) in inflammation. Receptor 1994; 4(1): 17-23.
[PMID: 8038702]

[128] WCRF/AICR. World Cancer Research Fund/American Institute for Cancer Research. Food, nutrition, physical activity, and the prevention of cancer: a global perspective 1994.

[129] DeVita VT, Lawrence TS, Rosenberg SA. Cancer: principles & practice of oncology: primer of the molecular biology of cancer. Lippincott Williams & Wilkins. 2012.

[130] Organization Mondiale de la santé. WHO traditional medicine strategy 2002-2005. World Health Organization 2002.

SUBJECT INDEX

www.ingramcontent.com/pod-product-compliance
Lightning Source LLC
Chambersburg PA
CBHW041706210326
41598CB00007B/549